HEMATOLOGIC PROBLEMS

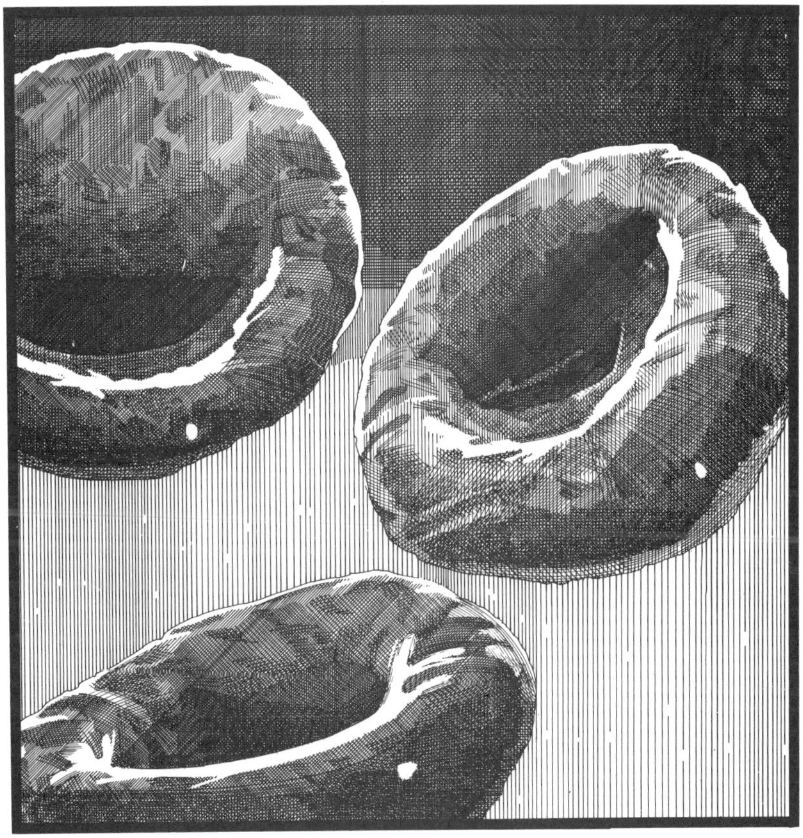

NurseReview™

Staff for this section

Book Editor
Kathy Goldberg

Editors
Catherine E. Harold
June Norris

Clinical Editor
Joan E. Mason, RN, EdM

Drug Information Managers
George J. Blake, MS, RPh
Larry Neil Gever, RPh, PharmD

Designer
Lynn Foulk Purvis

Illustrators
Julia DeVito, Dan Fione, Robert Jackson

Project Coordinator
Aline S. Miller

Production Coordinators
Maureen B. Carmichael, Elizabeth B. Kiselev

Editorial Services Manager
David R. Moreau

Editorial Services Supervisor
Edith McMahon

Copy Editors
Nick Anastasio, Keith de Pinho, Diane M. Labus, Doris Weinstock, Debra Young

Art Production Manager
Robert Perry

Typography Manager
David C. Kosten

Typography Assistants
Alicia Dempsey, Brenda Mayer, Diane Paluba, Nancy Wirs

Senior Production Manager
Deborah C. Meiris

Assistant Production Managers
Lisa Weiss, T.A. Landis

Clinical Consultants for this section

A. Bruce Campbell, PhD, MD
Hematologist/Oncologist, Scripps Memorial Hospitals, LaJolla and Encinitas, California

Christina Kasprisin, RN, MS
Quality Attainment Coordinator, Saint Francis Hospital, Tulsa, Oklahoma

NRT10-010789

Library of Congress Cataloging-in-Publication Data

Hematologic problems.
(NurseReview)
Includes bibliographies and index.
1. Blood—Diseases—Nursing. 2. Hematology. I. Series. [DNLM: 1. Hematologic Diseases—nursing. WY 152.5 H487]
RC633.H425 1988 616.1'5 87-33572
ISBN 0-87434-221-X(SC)

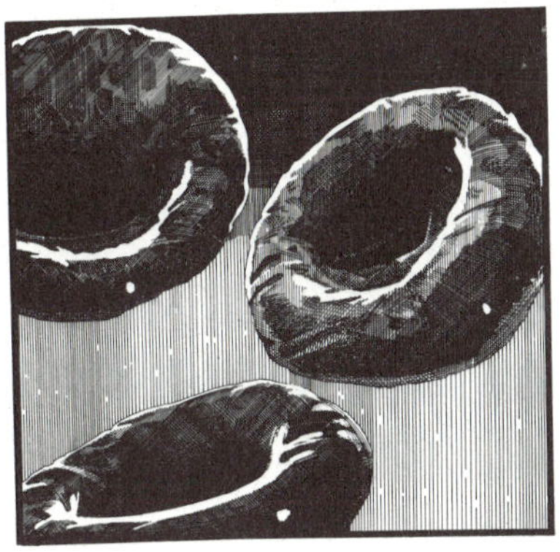

Contents

1 Introduction

Hematologic disorders can affect nearly every aspect of human life, escalating in some patients to life-threatening proportions. For patients affected by these disorders, your care must rest on a firm understanding of hematologic basics. Even when a patient's prognosis is poor, you can help him attain the best quality of life possible.

Hematologic Problems prepares you to meet this challenge. Written by recognized experts, the book serves as an up-to-date clinical reference. It reviews assessment techniques, diagnostic tests, treatments, and nursing interventions for anemias, polycythemias, leukemias, coagulopathies, and mononuclear phagocyte abnormalities.

Throughout the book you'll find information presented according to the nursing process, outlining your role every step of the way. Sample nursing care plans help you put nursing diagnoses into action by outlining patient goals, detailing nursing interventions, and specifying outcome criteria.

The first section, on patient assessment, includes one chapter on the history and physical examination and one chapter on diagnostic studies. The first chapter takes you through the process of taking a thorough health history—one that includes the patient's chief complaint, present illness, medical history, family history, and social history. You'll find that such factors as diet, medications, occupational hazards, and genetics may play an important role in hematologic disorders. The chapter then describes key signs and symptoms of hematologic disorders and provides a step-by-step guide to examining the patient.

The chapter on diagnostic tests reviews commonly performed blood tests, radiologic studies, lymph node biopsy, and bone marrow aspiration and biopsy. You'll learn how to prepare the patient for tests, participate in the procedures, care for the patient afterward, and understand the results. Numerous charts make normal test values and other important information easily accessible throughout the chapter.

The next chapter describes erythrocyte disorders. It begins with a concise review of blood cell development and includes a full-page chart showing how cells differentiate from pluripotent stem cells to specific blood cell types. You'll take a closer look at anemia, aplastic anemia, vitamin B_{12} deficiency, folic acid deficiency, iron deficiency, sideroblastic anemias, hereditary spherocytosis, sickle-cell anemia, thalassemias, and polycythemias.

The next chapter—on leukocyte disorders—reviews the four basic forms of leukemia. The text guides you through the proper nursing care, focusing on maintaining patient comfort and minimizing the adverse effects of therapy. Because many leukemia patients are children, you'll need special sensitivity to the emotional needs of both patient and family.

The section on hemorrhagic abnormalities includes chapters on congenital and acquired coagulation disorders. Congenital disorders covered in the section's first chapter include hemophilia, Von Willebrand's disease, hereditary hemorrhagic telangiectasia, and plate-

Introduction

let function disorders. A review of the normal coagulation process will help give you the underlying knowledge you'll need to care for these patients.

The other chapter in this section reviews such acquired coagulation disorders as immune thrombocytopenic purpura, disseminated intravascular coagulation, and vitamin K deficiency.

The next chapter covers lymphocyte disorders, including Hodgkin's disease, non-Hodgkin's lymphoma, mycosis fungoides, infectious mononucleosis, and acquired immune deficiency syndrome. You'll also find a general discussion of lymphocyte development, structure, and function.

The final chapter focuses on major disorders of plasma cells, monocytes, and macrophages. These include plasma cell myeloma, Waldenström's macroglobulinemia, histiocytosis, and Gaucher's disease. The chapter also provides basic information on plasma cells, immunoglobulins, monocytes, and macrophages.

Concluding with references and an index, **Hematologic Problems** promises to be an important and practical addition to your nursing library. Like all the other volumes in the NurseReview series, it provides a professional boost in today's challenging health care environment.

Patient Assessment: History Taking and Physical Examination

Regina M. Shannon-Bodnar, Oncology Clinical Nurse Specialist at University of Maryland Cancer Center, Baltimore, wrote this chapter. She received her MS in Anatomy from New York Medical College and MSN from Yale University School of Nursing, New Haven, Conn. She has also received certification in Oncology Nursing.

Organ groups make up most body systems. In contrast, the hematologic system contains the blood, the major body *fluid,* and the blood-forming sites, including bone marrow and lymph nodes. The blood delivers oxygen and nutrients to all tissues and removes wastes. Red blood cells transport hemoglobin, white blood cells fight infections throughout the body, and platelets stick to injured blood vessel walls to form hemostatic plugs. Because the hematologic system directly affects and reacts to every other system, any disorder of it can prove challenging to assess.

Continued on page 4

Hematologic system: Blood and blood-forming sites

The blood cells include erythrocytes (red blood cells), leukocytes (white blood cells), and thrombocytes (platelets). Leukocytes come in two types: granular (basophils, eosinophils, and neutrophils) and nongranular (lymphocytes and monocytes).

Hematopoiesis occurs primarily in the bone marrow. Red marrow produces most blood cells; yellow marrow, which is mainly fat, can revert to hematopoietic tissue if necessary.

The lymph nodes and lymphoid tissue in the small intestine, spleen, tonsils, and thymus produce lymphocytes. Lymph nodes aggregate in regions, including the neck, axillary, epitrochlear, thoracic, abdominal, inguinal, and popliteal nodes. The cisterna chyli, a saclike chamber which lies anterior to the vertebral column, receives lymph from the intestinal, lumbar, and descending intercostal trunks.

The liver and spleen destroy aged blood cells. The liver also synthesizes plasma proteins and some clotting factors.

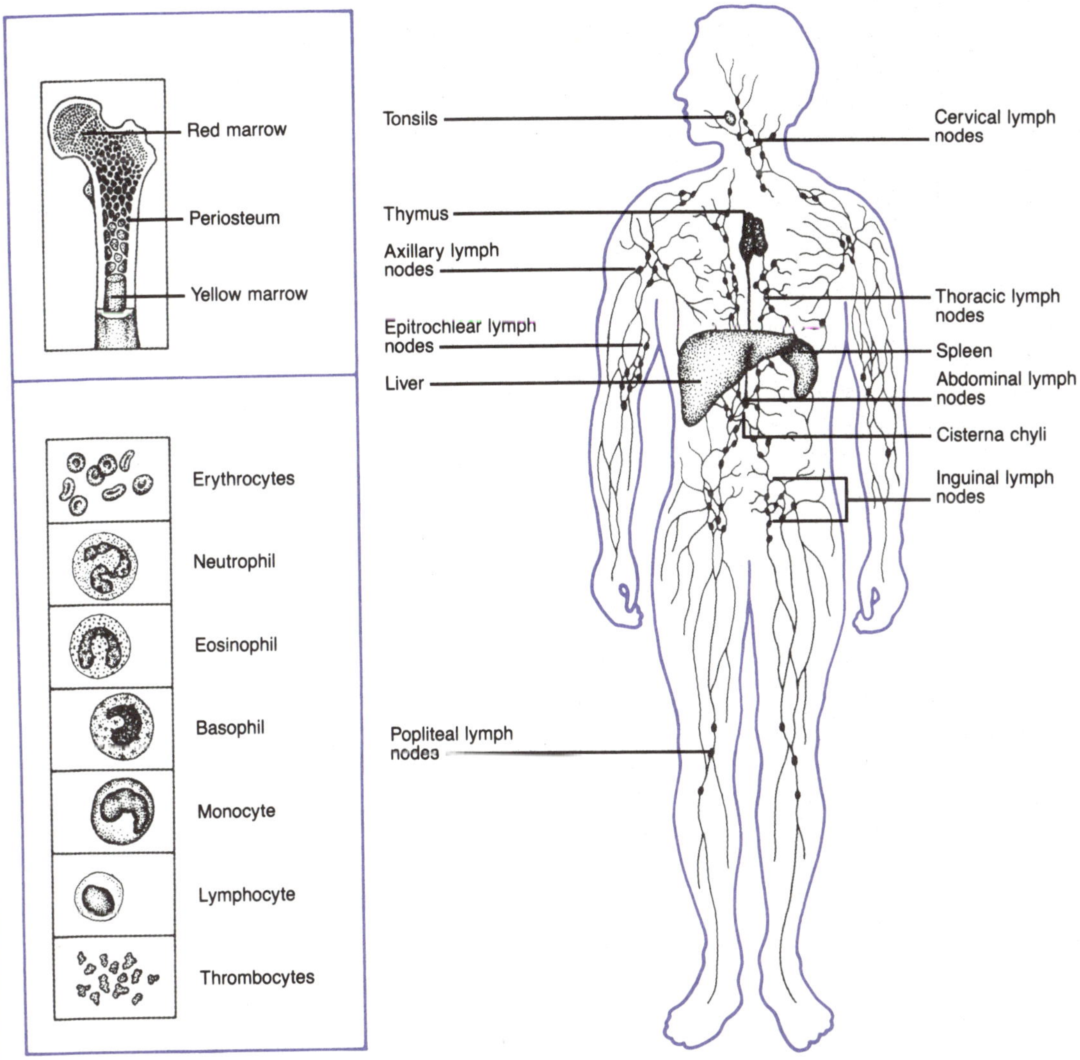

Patient Assessment

Continued

In this section, which includes Chapters 1 and 2, we'll review assessment techniques and diagnostic studies for the patient with hematologic problems.

Nursing history

A thorough health history serves as a major component in patient assessment. Here's an outline that will help you gather the necessary information. Use this information to guide your physical assessment.

In taking the history, ask open-ended questions to quickly identify specific concerns that need further investigation. Establish rapport with your patient to ensure accurate and complete responses. If possible, query the patient systematically to avoid overlooking important information. This can prove especially helpful if you have to conduct the interview in several short sessions because your patient's severely ill or your time's limited. Include the patient's diet, medication, and occupational histories, because these factors can play important roles in hematologic disorders.

Chief complaint

Ask the patient why he sought medical attention. Document the complaint in his own words. Because signs and symptoms from hematologic problems can appear in any body system, complaints will often be nonspecific: no energy, lightheadedness, nosebleeds. In themselves, such complaints may not prove diagnostic. But a complete nursing history may suggest a pattern that will lead you to suspect a hematologic disorder. For example, suppose your patient says he suffers shortness of breath, another nonspecific complaint. Without the complete history, you might concentrate on the patient's cardiovascular or respiratory system and overlook the possibility that his primary problem may be anemia.

If the patient complains about more than one problem, ask which bothers him the most. Concentrate on that complaint.

Present illness

Begin by obtaining the patient's biographic data. (See *Biographic data: Clues to risk factors.*) Then, ask the patient to give you a sign and symptom chronology. Be sure to obtain the following information about each sign and symptom:

- *onset.* When did it first occur? Did it appear suddenly or gradually?
- *incidence.* How often does it occur?
- *duration.* How long does it last?
- *manner.* Does it occur continuously or intermittently? If intermittently, how frequent and how long is each episode?
- *location.* Where does the patient feel it?
- *character.* What does it feel like? How severe is it?
- *precipitating conditions.* Does some activity bring it on?
- *aggravating/alleviating factors.* Does anything make it better or worse?
- *associated manifestations.* Do other signs or symptoms occur at the same time as the primary one?

Biographic data: Clues to risk factors

Record the patient's age, sex, marital status, occupation, education, religion, race, and ethnic background. These biographic factors provide clues to risk factors.

For example, hemophilia occurs almost exclusively in males, but females may carry the gene. Sickle cell anemia occurs primarily in blacks but also in persons with Mediterranean, Middle Eastern, or Asian ancestry. Vitamin B_{12} deficiency anemia (pernicious anemia) occurs most frequently in persons with a Northern European ancestry.

Patient Assessment

Minor problems: Easy to overlook

Sometimes a patient's health status changes so subtly that he may not notice it. Or he may judge such problems too minor to mention. But these problems could indicate an ineffective hematologic system. To uncover these easily overlooked symptoms, ask the following questions:
• Have you noticed increased bleeding after dental work or with routine flossing?
• Do you have frequent bruises, but can't remember their cause?
• (In female patients) Are your menstrual periods longer than usual? Do they occur more frequently? How regular are they? Has the menstrual flow changed? If so, how?
• Have you recently had a stiff neck? Any other aches?
• Do you have sores that are slow to heal?
• Have you experienced persistent colds, sore throats, or earaches lately?
• Have you lost your appetite? Have you recently lost weight without dieting? If so, how much?

Try to determine how the patient feels about his condition. Tailor your care to fit his perceptions. A worried patient may need more support, but an unconcerned one may need more patient teaching to promote compliance with therapy.

Be sure to collect data on your patient's general health status. Ask him whether he's suffered a recent illness. Could the present complaint be a new manifestation from a previously diagnosed illness? For example: in many cases, small cell lung cancer spreads to the bone marrow, causing fatigue and malaise. Occasionally, such viral illnesses as influenza and infectious mononucleosis can lead to hemolytic anemia. Also, an intervention for another condition could explain the present problem. Long-term antibiotic therapy for a respiratory or urinary tract infection, for example, can cause a blood disorder. Cancer therapies—chemotherapy, radiation therapy, and immunotherapy—can affect bone marrow. (See *Minor problems: Easy to overlook.*)

Medical history

Search the patient's medical history for clues to his present condition. Gather information on allergies (including drug reactions), immunizations, previously diagnosed illnesses (childhood and adult), past hospitalizations and surgeries, and current medications.

Look for past disorders, such as acute leukemia, Hodgkin's disease, and sarcoma, that required aggressive marrow-suppressive drug or radiation therapies. Also note tumors that have bone marrow-seeking tendencies, such as small cell lung cancer or lymphoma. Hepatitis and miliary tuberculosis can also cause bone marrow failure.

Find out whether your patient was ever hospitalized and why. Could a past surgical intervention now be causing a medical problem? A total or partial gastrectomy or lower ileum resection may contribute to vitamin and nutrient malabsorption resulting in anemia. A splenectomy places the patient at high risk for disseminated infection with encapsulated organisms. Immunosuppressive therapy predisposes organ transplant patients to several disorders, particularly lymphoreticular cancers.

Did the patient receive blood transfusions? If so, note how often and when he received them to assess his risk for contracting an infectious agent. Before March 1985, donated blood was not tested for human immunodeficiency virus (HIV), the causative agent in acquired immune deficiency syndrome (AIDS). Transfused blood products can also transmit non-A, non-B hepatitis, cytomegalovirus, malaria, and Epstein-Barr virus, associated with Burkitt's lymphoma.

Has the patient undergone radiation therapy? Such treatment may diminish blood cell production. Remember, ask about thymus radiation in childhood.

Document all medications—prescription and over-the-counter. The patient who suffers from seizures probably takes anticonvulsant drugs that suppress bone marrow. Antineoplastic drugs can cause secondary leukemia or bone marrow dysfunction. (See *Some drugs that affect the hematologic system,* pages 6 and 7.)

Continued on page 7

Patient Assessment

Some drugs that affect the hematologic system

Drug	Possible hematologic effects
ANALGESICS	
Aspirin	Inhibited platelet aggregation, prolonged bleeding time
Phenylbutazone	Bone marrow depression, hemolytic anemia, leukopenia
ANTIARRHYTHMICS	
Propranolol	Agranulocytosis, inhibited platelet function
Quinidine	Agranulocytosis, anemia, leukopenia, thrombocytopenia
ANTICONVULSANTS	
Carbamazepine	Anemia, leukopenia, thrombocytopenia
Mephenytoin	Agranulocytosis, leukopenia
Phenacemide	Agranulocytosis, aplastic anemia
Phenytoin	Agranulocytosis, leukopenia, thrombocytopenia
ANTIGOUT AGENT	
Colchicine	Aplastic anemia, agranulocytosis, nonthrombocytic purpura
ANTIHYPERTENSIVES	
Captopril	Agranulocytosis, leukopenia, pancytopenia
Methyldopa	Hemolytic anemia, reversible granulocytopenia, thrombocytopenia
ANTI-INFLAMMATORY AGENTS	
Ibuprofen	Prolonged bleeding time
Indomethacin	Agranulocytosis, aplastic anemia, hemolytic anemia, iron deficiency anemia, leukopenia, thrombocytopenia
Naproxen	Prolonged bleeding time
ANTIMICROBIAL AGENTS	
Amphotericin B	Anemia, granulocytopenia
Chloramphenicol	Aplastic anemia, thrombocytopenia
Chloroquine	Agranulocytosis, hemolytic anemia
Penicillin	Eosinophilia, hemolytic anemia, leukopenia, thrombocytopenia
Quinine	Agranulocytosis, hemolytic anemia, hypoprothrombinemia, thrombocytopenia
Sulfisoxazole	Agranulocytosis, aplastic anemia, hemolytic anemia, leukopenia, thrombocytopenia
Co-trimoxazole	Agranulocytosis, anemia, aplastic anemia, hemolytic anemia, leukopenia, thrombocytopenia
DIURETICS	
Chlorothiazide	Agranulocytosis, aplastic anemia, leukopenia, thrombocytopenia
Furosemide	Agranulocytosis, leukopenia, thrombocytopenia
GOLD SALTS	
Auranofin	Agranulocytosis, aplastic anemia, eosinophilia, leukopenia, thrombocytopenia
Aurothioglucose	Same as above
IMMUNOSUPPRESSANTS	
Azathioprine	Anemia, bone marrow depression, leukopenia, thrombocytopenia

continued

Patient Assessment

Some drugs that affect the hematologic system—*continued*

Drug	Possible hematologic effects
PSYCHOTHERAPEUTICS	
Chlorpromazine	Agranulocytosis, transient leukopenia
Haloperidol	Leukocytosis, transient leukopenia
Lithium	Leukocytosis
Thioridazine	Agranulocytosis, transient leukopenia
THYROID HORMONAL AGENTS	
Methimazole	Agranulocytosis, granulocytopenia, leukopenia, thrombocytopenia
Propylthiouracil	Agranulocytosis, leukopenia, thrombocytopenia

Nursing history—*continued*

Erythrocyte development relies on dietary iron, folic acid, and vitamin B_{12}. Deficiencies in these and other vitamins and minerals may provide diagnostic clues. So be sure to obtain a complete diet history.

Family history
Some hematologic conditions involve genetic components. So a thorough family history's important. Understanding immediate family members' health status may help fine tune the patient's complaint and establish familial patterns. Ask about deceased family members, recording age at death and cause.

Note any inheritable hematologic disorders and plot them on a family genogram to determine the inheritance risk. The most common are:
- *hemophilia.* This X-linked recessive bleeding disorder, resulting from specific clotting factor deficiencies, occurs almost exclusively in males; females may carry the gene.
- *Von Willebrand's disease.* This autosomal dominant bleeding disorder, resulting from moderate clotting Factor VIII deficiency and impaired platelet function, affects males and females equally.
- *sickle cell anemia.* This chronic hemolytic anemia, characterized by a defective hemoglobin molecule (hemoglobin S), occurs primarily in blacks. Homozygous inheritance causes a severe disorder; heterozygous inheritance causes sickle cell trait, generally an asymptomatic condition.
- *thalassemia.* This chronic hemolytic anemia group, characterized by defective hemoglobin synthesis, occurs primarily in persons with Mediterranean ancestry. Homozygous inheritance causes a severe form; heterozygous inheritance's usually asymptomatic.

Congenital aplastic anemias, such as that which occurs in Fanconi's anemia, may also have a genetic origin.

Note the familial patterns in such hematologic cancers as leukemia, Hodgkin's disease, and non-Hodgkin's lymphoma. Experts suspect that viruses may be at least partly responsible for these cancers. Genetics may also play a role in leukemia. A monozygotic twin has a 20% to 25% chance to develop leukemia if his twin has it, particulary in infancy. Data also link an increased leukemia incidence to such chromosomal abnormalities as Down's and Klinefel-

Continued on page 8

Patient Assessment

Nursing history—*continued*

ter's syndromes and to syndromes accompanied by chromosomal fragility, including Bloom's syndrome and Fanconi's anemia, the syndrome also associated with aplastic anemia.

Social history

Life-style and occupation may adversely affect hematologic function. Remember, the patient may be reluctant to discuss certain habits or his life-style. Developing trust between you and your patient can increase cooperation. Alcoholism can cause folic acid deficiency anemia because excessive alcohol intake interferes with folic acid metabolism, disordering erythroid cell maturation. Also, the poor diet common in alcoholics may lack sufficient folic acid. AIDS occurs primarily among homosexual and bisexual men, especially those with multiple sexual partners. Anal intercourse and other sexual practices involving exposure to blood or semen spread the disease. Sharing infected I.V. needles also transmits AIDS, so I.V. drug abusers also risk contracting it. AIDS has also occurred among heterosexuals who have sexual relations with AIDS patients or AIDS carriers.

Exposure to certain hazardous compounds and chemicals may cause bone marrow dysfunction, especially leukemia. So be sure to gather a comprehensive occupational history. (See *Some occupational haz-*

Some occupational hazards

The following agents have been implicated in hematologic disorders.

Agent	Occupation	Disorder
Benzene	• Chemical industry workers • Glue and varnish makers • Painters • Plastics factory workers • Rubber cement makers • Rubber tire manufacturing workers • Shoemakers • Shoe manufacturing workers	Aplastic anemia, leukemia
Epichlorohydrin	• Chemical industry workers	Aplastic anemia, leukemia
Ethylene oxide	• Hospital workers • Research laboratory workers	Aplastic anemia, leukemia
Insecticides	• Farmers • Horticulturists	Leukemia, lymphoma
Ionizing radiation	• Health care workers • Luminous dial painters • Radiographers • Radiologists • Uranium miners	Aplastic anemia, leukemia, lymphoma
Thorium dioxide	• Ceramic industry workers • Chemical industry workers • Gas mantle makers • Incandescent lamp makers • Metal refiners • Nuclear reactor workers • Steel workers • Vacuum tube makers	Aplastic anemia, leukemia, lymphoma
Vinyl chloride	• Plastics factory workers • Vinyl chloride polymerization plant workers	Leukemia, lymphoma

Patient Assessment

ards.) Ask about ionizing radiation exposure. Experts have uncovered a strong link between ionizing radiation and aplastic anemia and hematologic cancers. Also ask the patient about his military service. Vietnam veterans exposed to Agent Orange show a higher-than-normal leukemia and lymphoma incidence. Although the data remain controversial, exposure to this chemical may be responsible.

Key signs and symptoms

Although the general signs and symptoms often prove nonspecific and difficult to assess in hematologic disorders, certain key signs and symptoms can alert you to these conditions. Remember, they'll vary according to each disorder and stem cell line. Look for these:

Abnormal bleeding
Excessive blood loss may cause anemia. The patient who reports bruises from minimal pressure or slight bumps, prolonged bleeding after teeth cleaning, or bleeding for no apparent reason may suffer a clotting mechanism deficiency. Besides hereditary conditions, such a deficiency can arise from drug therapy that produces bone marrow depression.

Fatigue and weakness
These can vary in severity according to the disorder. Fatigue and weakness accompanying moderate exertion may mean moderate anemia. Extreme or constant fatigue and weakness might indicate severe anemia, leukemia, lymphoma, or plasma cell myeloma.

Fever
Fever may indicate infection. Frequently recurring fevers may indicate rapid cell proliferation, such as that which occurs in leukemia or lymphomas. Hodgkin's disease, in particular, has the characteristic Pel-Ebstein fever pattern, in which fever lasting several days alternates with afebrile periods.

Lymphadenopathy
Swollen lymph nodes may mean inflammation from infection or the elevated lymphocyte production from certain leukemias. Primary lymphatic tumors aren't usually painful, but enlarged lymph nodes may accompany Hodgkin's disease.

Joint and bone pain
Pain in the knees, hands, or wrists may indicate hemarthrosis (blood in the joint), stemming from a bleeding disorder. Aching bones may result from the pressure caused by expanding bone marrow from acute myelocytic leukemia. Joint pain may result from direct invasion by such diseases as leukemias and plasma cell myeloma.

Physical examination

Because a hematologic disorder can involve almost every body system, be sure to perform a complete physical examination.

Vital signs can provide important clues. Take the patient's temperature. Frequent fevers can indicate a poorly functioning immune system. Subnormal temperatures most often occur with infections from gram-negative organisms. Note the heart rate. The heart may pump harder or faster to compensate for a decreased oxygen supply

Continued on page 10

Patient Assessment

Physical examination—*continued*

resulting from anemia or decreased blood volume from bleeding. This can cause tachycardia, palpitations, or dysrhythmias. Check respirations. The body's attempt to meet its oxygen needs could result in pronounced tachypnea. Measure blood pressure with the patient lying, sitting, and standing. Check for orthostatic hypotension, as well as hypotension possibly caused by septicemia or hypovolemia.

Finally, assess your patient's level of consciousness. Impairment may result from hypoxia, fever, or even an active intracranial hemorrhage. Be alert for critical changes that require the doctor's immediate attention. Look for the impairment's cause only after you've initiated intervention and stabilized the patient hemodynamically. Next, concentrate on areas most relevant to a hematologic disorder:
- skin
- mucous membranes
- nails
- eyes
- lymph nodes
- liver
- spleen.

See *Review of systems* for your complete examination.

Inspection

Skin and mucous membranes. Check your patient's skin color; it directly reflects body fluid composition. Note any pallor, cyanosis, or jaundice. Decreased hemoglobin content can cause pallor. Cyanosis results from excessive deoxygenated hemoglobin in cutaneous blood vessels, a condition caused by hypoxia, which appears in some anemias. Cyanosis or pallor in a patient's fingers or toes may result from Raynaud's phenomenon, seen in some autoimmune diseases. Jaundice may be caused by hemolysis from sickle cell anemia.

Examine the patient's face, conjunctivae, hands, and feet for plethora (ruddy color), which appears in polycythemia. Inspect for erythema, which may mean local inflammation or fever. Pay particular attention to the skin over your patient's lymph nodes. Note any color abnormalities. Nodes covered by red-streaked skin suggest a lymphatic disorder, including acute lymphadenitis. With lymphadenitis, also look for an obvious infection site.

Look for jaundice in the patient's mucous membranes and skin, being sure to observe him in the daylight. Incandescent light can mask yellow color. With dark-skinned patients, inspect the buccal mucosa, palms, and soles for a yellowish tinge. For an edematous patient, examine the inner forearm for jaundice. An elevated bilirubin level may appear secondary to increased erythrocyte hemolysis—either acquired or hereditary. *Note:* Excessive carrot or yellow-vegetable intake may cause yellow skin but will not change sclerae or mucous membrane color.

If you suspect a blood clotting abnormality, check the patient's skin for purpuric lesions. These usually result from thrombocytopenia and can vary in size. With dark-skinned patients, check the oral mucosa or conjunctivae for petechiae or ecchymoses. As the body

Continued on page 12

Patient Assessment

Review of systems

If you uncover these findings during the physical examination, suspect these possible hematologic causes.

System/Finding	Possible cause
NEUROLOGIC	
Confusion	• Cancerous or infectious process involving the brain, severe anemia
Headache	• Anemia, brain hemorrhage from thrombocytopenia or other bleeding disorders, brain invasion or compression from leukemia, lymphoma, or infection, polycythemia
Impairment of consciousness	• Increased intracranial pressure from hemorrhage or tumor, polycythemia, severe anemia
Lightheadedness	• Anorexia from anemia
Paresthesia	• Hematologic cancer, vitamin B_{12} deficiency anemia, polycythemia, vincristine therapy
EYE, EAR, NOSE, THROAT	
Anosmia	• Vitamin B_{12} deficiency anemia
Bleeding gums or oral mucosa	• Polycythemia, thrombocytopenia, other bleeding disorders
Blindness	• Retinal hemorrhages from anemia or thrombocytopenia
Conjunctival pallor	• Reduced hemoglobin
Epistaxis	• Bleeding disorders, polycythemia
Jaundiced sclera	• Excessive hemolysis leading to bile pigment accumulation
Smooth tongue	• Iron deficiency anemia, vitamin B_{12} deficiency anemia, or other vitamin deficiencies
Sore tongue	• Vitamin B_{12} deficiency anemia
Ulcerated tongue or oral mucosa	• Leukemia, neutropenia
Vertigo, tinnitus	• Polycythemia, severe anemia
Visual disturbances	• Anemia, polycythemia
CARDIOPULMONARY	
Angina pectoris	• Anemia
Dyspnea	• Anemia, lymphoma, polycythemia
Murmurs	• Anemia
Tachycardia possibly with palpations	• Anemia, polycythemia
GASTROINTESTINAL	
Abdominal pain	• Acute hemolysis, allergic purpura, intestinal obstruction by lymphoma, retroperitoneal bleeding, sickle cell anemia
Anorexia	• Nonspecific

System/Finding	Possible cause
GASTROINTESTINAL continued	
Diarrhea	• Malabsorption from small bowel lymphoma, vitamin B_{12} deficiency anemia
Dysphagia	• Chronic iron deficiency anemia leading to mucous membrane atrophy
Hematemesis, melena	• Thrombocytopenia, other bleeding disorders
Hepatomegaly, splenomegaly	• Hemolytic anemia, leukemia, lymphoma, polycythemia
Pain with defecation	• Neutropenia
Pica	• Iron deficiency anemia
GENITOURINARY	
Amenorrhea	• Nonspecific
Hematuria	• Bleeding disorders
Impotence, bladder dysfunction	• Spinal cord or peripheral nerve damage from hematologic cancers
Menorrhagia	• Bleeding disorders, iron deficiency
Red urine	• Intravascular hemolysis, diet high in beets in iron-deficient patients
INTEGUMENTARY	
Cyanosis	• Methemoglobinemia
Dry, coarse skin	• Iron deficiency anemia
Ecchymosis	• Coagulation defects
Itching	• Chronic lymphatic leukemia, Hodgkin's disease, lymphoma, polycythemia
Jaundice	• Hemolytic anemia, liver involvement, vitamin B_{12} deficiency anemia, sickle cell anemia
Pallor	• Reduced hemoglobin
Petechiae, purpura	• Blood vessel abnormalities, leukemia, platelet abnormalities
Plethora	• Polycythemia
MUSCULOSKELETAL	
Arthritis, arthralgia	• Acute leukemia, gout (from increased uric acid production caused by hematologic cancers or hemolytic anemia), hemarthroses from bleeding disorders, sickle cell anemia
Back pain	• Hemolytic reactions
Bone pain	• Congenital hemolytic anemias, such as sickle cell anemia; hematologic cancers
Leg edema (lower extremities)	• Enlarged lymph nodes causing venous or lymphatic obstruction
Leg ulcers	• Sickle cell anemia
Sternal tenderness	• Anemia, leukemia, plasma cell myeloma

Patient Assessment

Skin signs: A glossary

Petechiae. Tiny purplish, red round spots that appear on skin and mucous membranes resulting from intradermal or submucosal hemorrhage.

Ecchymosis. A blue or purplish patch, larger than a petechia, from a ruptured blood vessel; commonly called a bruise.

Purpura. General term for several hemorrhagic states marked by patches of purplish discoloration resulting from extravasation of blood into the skin and mucous membranes; includes ecchymoses and petechiae.

Physical examination—*continued*

resorbs blood, the skin color changes from yellow to yellow green, which is difficult to detect in dark-skinned individuals. Be sure to inspect for abnormalities such as telangiectases and note their location. (See *Skin signs: A glossary.*)

Check your patient's skin for dryness and coarseness, indicating iron deficiency anemia. Ask him whether his skin itches. Itching (pruritus) can indicate Hodgkin's disease, chronic lymphocytic leukemia, or polycythemia vera.

Check skin integrity. Make a note if you find any infection signs—abnormal temperature, wound drainage, poor wound healing, or ulceration.

Look at your patient's mucous membranes, particularly the gingival structures. Be alert for bleeding, redness, swelling, or ulceration. These signs may indicate leukemia. A smooth tongue can signify vitamin B_{12} deficiency or iron deficiency anemia. An ulcerated tongue may mean leukemia or neutropenia. Fluffy white patches scattered throughout the oral cavity indicate Candida, a fungal infection. Hairy leukoplakia, a lacey white plaque found typically on the buccal mucosa, appears with AIDS.

Nails. Inspect the patient's nails and note any abnormalities. Longitudinal striation can indicate anemia. Koilonychia (spoon nail) characterizes iron deficiency anemia. Platyonychia (abnormally broad or flat nails) may precede koilonychia development. Nail clubbing indicates chronic hypoxia, which can result from such hematologic disorders as anemia.

Eyes. Inspect your patient's eyes for jaundice. Sclerae with a yellowish tinge can indicate an accumulation of bile pigment from excessive hemolysis. Retinal hemorrhages and exudates, observable with an ophthalmoscope, suggest severe anemia and thrombocytopenia.

Lymph nodes. Note any obvious enlargements or redness.

Liver and spleen. Inspect the abdominal area for enlargement, distention, and asymmetry, possibly indicating a tumor. Hepatomegaly and splenomegaly may result from congestion caused by cell overproduction, as in polycythemia or leukemia, or excessive cell destruction, as in hemolytic anemia.

Auscultation

With the patient lying down, auscultate the abdomen before palpation and percussion so you don't alter bowel sounds. Listen for loud, high-pitched tinkling sounds, indicating intestinal obstruction in its early stages. Lymphoma is a hematologic cause of such obstruction. Next, concentrate on auscultating the liver and spleen. Listen carefully over both organs for friction rubs—grating sounds that fluctuate with respiration. These sounds usually indicate inflammation of the organ's peritoneal covering. Liver friction rubs also may mean primary or metastatic (infiltrative) tumor. Splenic friction rubs also suggest infarction and inflammation.

Percussion

This procedure helps detect tumors and determine liver and spleen size. Percuss all four quadrants and compare your findings.

Patient Assessment

Palpating neck nodes

To palpate the preauricular nodes, position your fingers as shown here.

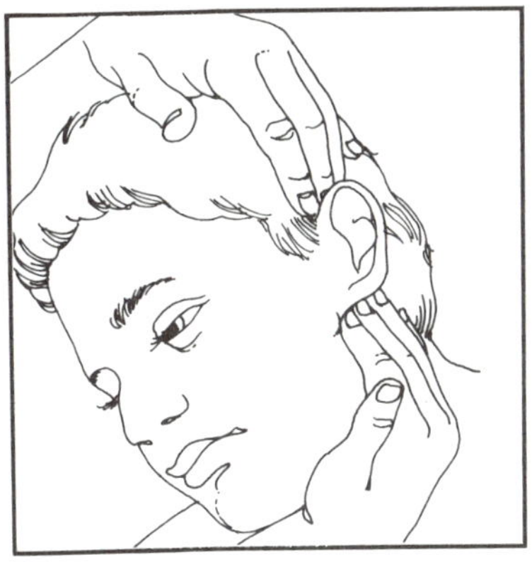

To palpate the submandibular, submental, and cervical nodes, position your fingers as shown here. Palpate over the mandibular surface and continue moving up and down the entire neck. Flex the head forward or to the side being examined to relax the tissues and make enlarged nodes more palpable.

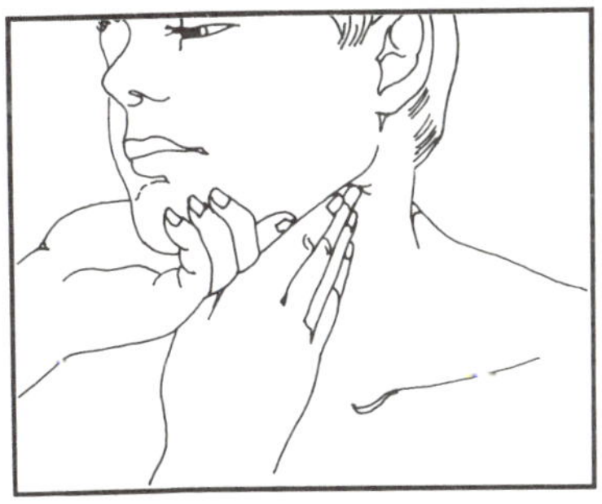

To palpate the supraclavicular nodes, first encourage your patient to relax, so his clavicles drop. Flex his head slightly forward to relax the soft tissues of his anterior neck. Then, hook your index finger over the clavicle lateral to the sternocleidomastoid muscle. Rotate your finger deeply into this area to feel these nodes.

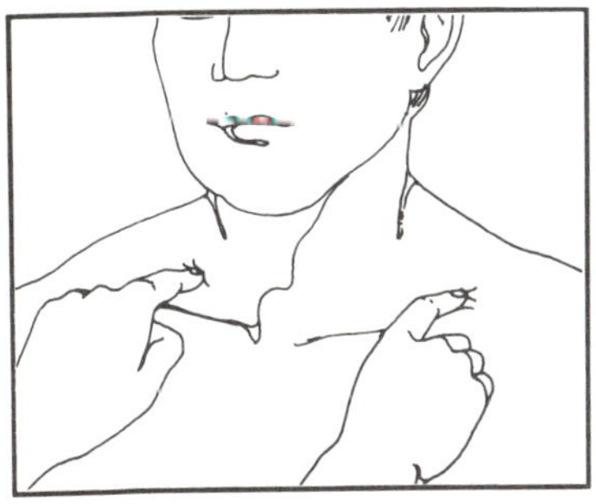

Palpating axillary nodes

To palpate the axillary nodes, gently press the soft tissues against the chest wall and the muscles surrounding the axilla (the pectoral muscles, latissimus dorsi, subscapularis, and serratus anterior muscles).

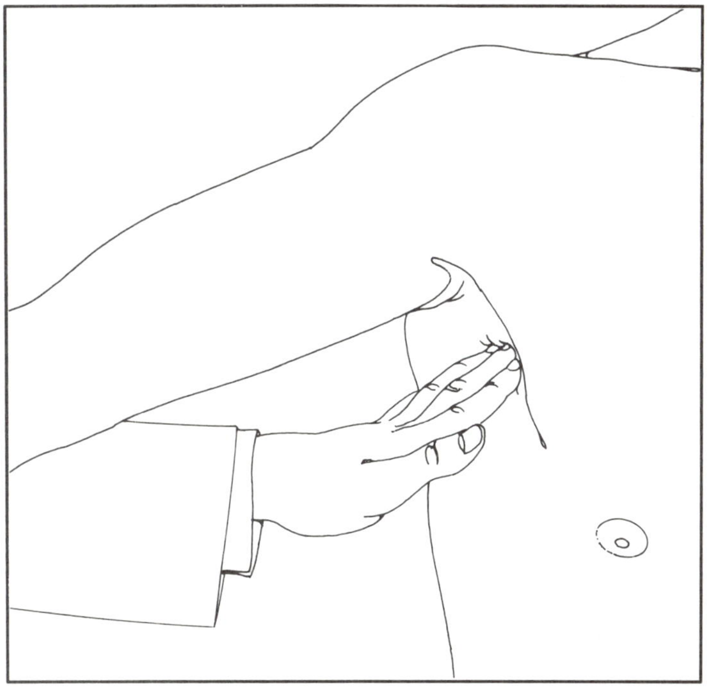

The normal liver sounds dull. To determine the organ's approximate size, percuss for its upper and lower borders at the mid-clavicular line. To determine medial extension, percuss to the mid-sternal landmark.

The spleen also sounds dull. You should percuss from the mid-axillary toward the midline. The average-size spleen will lie near the 8th, 9th, or 10th intercostal space.

You might want to mark liver and spleen borders with a pen for later reference when palpating these organs.

Palpation

Lymph nodes. Palpate your patient's neck, axillary, epitrochlear, and inguinal lymph nodes, moving skin over each area with your finger pads.

When palpating nodes in the neck, make sure the patient is sitting. (See *Palpating neck nodes.*) He should remain sitting or lie down when you palpate his axillary nodes. For the right axilla, ask the patient to relax his right arm. Use your nondominant hand to support it. Put your other hand as high in his right axilla as possible. Palpate against the chest wall for the lateral, anterior, posterior, central, and subclavian nodes. Repeat the procedure for the patient's left axilla. (See *Palpating axillary nodes.*) For the epitrochlear nodes, palpate his elbow's medial area. For the inguinal nodes, palpate below the inguinal ligament and along the upper saphenous vein.

Continued on page 14

Patient Assessment

Physical examination—*continued*

As you palpate all nodes, note their location, size, tenderness, texture (hard, soft, firm), and fixation (moveable or fixed). For each node group, note the symmetry.

Palpable nodes and lymphedema may indicate a lymphatic disorder. Enlarged or tender nodes suggest current or previous inflammation. Hard or fixed nodes may suggest a tumor. General lymphadenopathy can indicate an inflammatory or cancerous condition.

As you palpate nodes, you may discover sternal tenderness. This problem occurs with cell packing in the marrow from anemia, leukemia, and immunoproliferative disorders.

Liver and spleen. Lightly palpate all four abdominal quadrants to distinguish tender sites and muscle guarding. Deeper palpation helps delineate abdominal organs and masses. Always palpate tender areas last.

To palpate the liver, place your left hand underneath the patient at the 11th and 12th ribs and press forward. With your right hand, press gently in and up on the patient's right abdomen below the lower border where you determined liver dullness with percussion. Ask the patient to take a deep breath. You should feel the liver's edge as it descends downward toward your finger tips, with the increase in intrathoracic pressure and volume. Note the liver's contour and surface. A normal liver's edge feels smooth, regular, and firm.

A difficult procedure, accurate liver palpation can depend on the patient's size, the patient's present comfort level, and whether fluid's present. If necessary, repeat the procedure, checking your hand position and the pressure you exert.

To palpate the spleen, reach over the patient and place your left hand beneath the lower left rib cage. Press forward gently. With your right hand, press in toward the spleen, where you have approximated its position with percussion just below the left costal margin. Be sure to allow enough space between your hand and the rib cage border for sufficient mobility. Ask the patient to take a deep breath. The spleen should descend to meet your fingertips. You may need to position the patient on his right side and flex his hips and knees to facilitate splenic palpation. This position brings the spleen forward and to the right. Remember, you can only feel a spleen that's enlarged approximately three times its original size. You won't be able to palpate a normal or slightly enlarged spleen.

As you palpate the liver and spleen, watch your patient carefully for discomfort when you withdraw your hand. Look for facial grimacing, muscle guarding, and knee flexion. Pay attention to your patient's complaints; discomfort can indicate various disorders.

Diagnostic Studies: Patient Teaching, Preparation, and Nursing Care

Cecilia E. Shaw, who wrote this chapter, is Nurse Manager and Research Coordinator for Hematology Oncology Associates, Inc., Tulsa, Okla. She received her BSN from the University of Oklahoma, Norman. She is also a certified medical-surgical and oncology nurse.

The patient with a known or suspected hematologic disorder usually will need to undergo various diagnostic tests to pinpoint his problem. These tests directly examine the blood, the bone marrow, and the lymph nodes.

In this chapter, we'll discuss specific diagnostic procedures—blood tests, radiologic studies, lymph node biopsy, and bone marrow aspiration and needle biopsy—that assess for hematologic problems.

Most tests for hematologic disorders require venipuncture to obtain blood samples. Although the procedure's probably routine for you, venipuncture can cause patient anxiety. Some patients fear that the needle stick will cause pain, especially if the vein proves hard to find. Others may faint at the sight of blood or worry that the test will yield abnormal results.

You'll prepare the patient for testing and provide postprocedure care. Keep the following considerations in mind when caring for a patient undergoing tests to assess for a hematologic disorder:
- Make sure the patient knows the test's name and its purpose.
- Remind your patient not to eat or drink before the procedure, if indicated by doctor's orders and hospital policy.

Continued on page 16

Color-top collection tubes: A guide

Here's a handy reference guide to collection tubes used for hematologic studies.

RED

Red-top *tubes contain no additives. Draw volume may be 2 to 20 ml. These tubes are used for tests performed on serum samples.*
- ABO blood typing
- Antibody screening test
- Antiglobulin
- Antinuclear antibodies
- Antistreptolysin-O test
- Bilirubin
- Cold agglutinins
- Complement assays
- Cross matching
- Direct antiglobulin
- Ferritin
- Folic acid
- Haptoglobin
- Immune complex assays
- Immunoglobulins G, A, and M
- Lactic dehydrogenase
- Leukoagglutinins
- Plasma antidepressants
- Plasma LH
- Prothrombin consumption time
- Rh typing
- Vitamin B_{12}

GRAY

Gray-top *tubes contain a glycolytic inhibitor (such as sodium fluoride, powdered oxalate, or glycolytic/microbial inhibitor). Draw volume may be 3 to 10 ml. These tubes are used most often for glucose determinations in serum or plasma samples.*
- Anti-DNA antibodies

LAVENDER

Lavender-top *tubes contain edetate. Draw volume may be 2 to 10 ml. These tubes are used for tests performed on whole blood samples.*
- ABO blood typing
- Anti-DNA antibodies
- Erythrocyte sedimentation rate
- Glucagon
- Glycosylated hemoglobin
- G6PD
- Heinz bodies
- Hematocrit
- Hemoglobin electrophoresis
- Lipoprotein phenotyping
- Plasma renin activity
- Platelet count
- Platelet survival
- Pyruvate kinase
- Red blood cell (RBC) count
- Red cell indices
- Reticulocyte count
- Rh typing
- Sickle-cell test (hemoglobin S)
- Total hemoglobin
- Unstable hemoglobins
- White blood cell (WBC) count
- WBC differential

BLACK

Black-top *tubes contain sodium oxalate. Draw volume may be 2.7 or 4.5 ml. These tubes are used for coagulation studies performed on plasma samples.*
- Plasma vitamin C

BLUE

Blue-top *tubes contain sodium citrate and citric acid. Draw volume may be 2.7 or 4.5 ml. These tubes are used for coagulation studies requiring plasma samples.*
- Activated partial thromboplastin time
- Euglobulin lysis time
- Fibrinogen
- Hemoglobin derivatives
- One-stage assay: Extrinsic coagulation system
- One-stage assay: Intrinsic coagulation system
- Plasminogen
- Platelet aggregation
- Prothrombin time
- Thrombin time

GREEN (heparinized)

Green-top *tubes contain heparin (sodium, lithium, or ammonium). Draw volume may be 2 to 15 ml. These tubes are used for tests performed on plasma samples.*
- Erythropoietic porphyrins
- Lymphocyte transformation tests
- Osmotic fragility
- RBC survival time
- T- and B-lymphocyte counts

Diagnostic Studies

Continued

- Use the correct collection tube for tests requiring specific preservatives or anticoagulants. (See *Color-top collection tubes: A guide,* page 15.) That way, you'll avoid unnecessary cost and patient anxiety caused by a repeated needle stick.
- Use proper technique to avoid unnecessary exposure to agents that may cause infectious disease.

Blood tests

Analysis of peripheral blood samples provides diagnostic information useful in selecting follow-up tests. Blood test results also help guide therapy—for example, by indicating the patient's response to radiation therapy and chemotherapy.

(*Note:* The normal laboratory values listed in the following sections may differ slightly from those given in your hospital's laboratory manual.)

Complete blood count (CBC)
The complete blood count includes the red blood cell (RBC) count, total hemoglobin concentration, hematocrit, red cell indices, white blood cell (WBC) count, and WBC differential. It commonly includes a platelet count as well. The CBC describes the quantity, type, form, and structure of each blood element.

RBC count. Also known as the erythrocyte count, the RBC count measures the number of RBCs in a microliter (cubic millimeter) of whole blood. This test supplies values used to compute the red cell indices, which reveal RBC size and hemoglobin content. It can also verify findings from other hematologic tests used to diagnose anemia and polycythemia.

Normal RBC values vary with age, sex, sample, and laboratory method. The following ranges serve as a guide:
- Men—4.5 to 6.2 million/μl
- Women—4.2 to 5.4 million/μl
- Children—4.6 to 4.8 million/μl.

Normal hemoglobin concentration: Age and sex variations

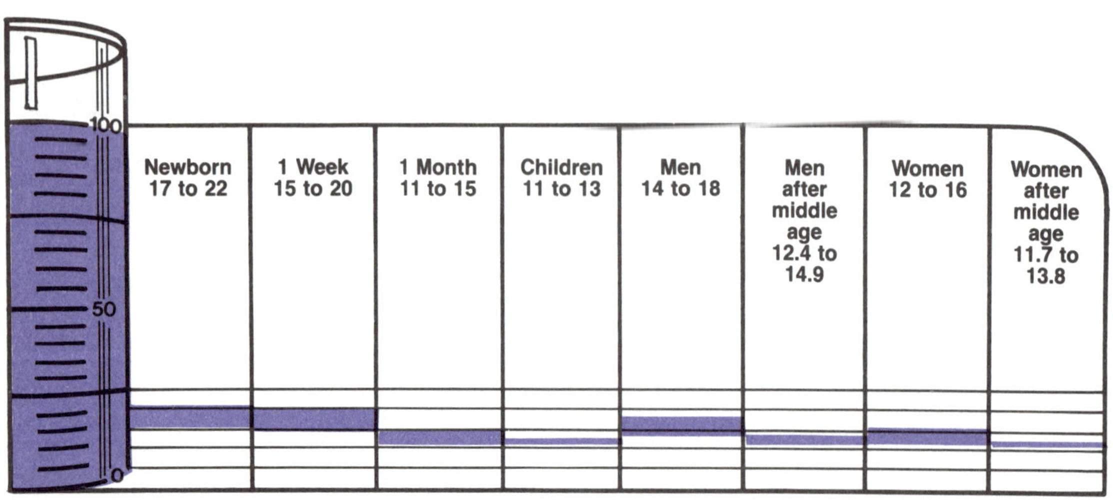

KEY: Hemoglobin g/dl

Diagnostic Studies

Decreased red blood cell count: What it suggests

A below-normal red blood cell (RBC) count may reflect any of the following abnormalities:
- insufficient RBC production from bone marrow dysfunction or deficiency of an essential hemopoietic factor
- increased RBC destruction from an intrinsic cell defect caused by such disorders as hereditary spherocytosis and thalassemia or such extrinsic factors as trauma or infection
- increased RBC loss from bleeding disorders or hemorrhage.

A depressed RBC count may indicate anemia, fluid overload, recent hemorrhage, or leukemia. An elevated RBC count may reflect dehydration, polycythemia (primary or secondary), or acute poisoning.

Total hemoglobin concentration. The red cell's major component, hemoglobin contains *heme,* a complex molecule of iron and porphyrin that gives blood its color, and *globin,* a simple protein. Hemoglobin delivers oxygen from the lungs to the cells and buffers carbon dioxide formed during metabolic activity.

The hemoglobin test measures the grams of hemoglobin in a deciliter (100 ml) of whole blood. This measurement helps indicate the severity of anemia or polycythemia. It also supplies values used to calculate mean corpuscular hemoglobin (MCH) and mean corpuscular hemoglobin concentration (MCHC). Hemoglobin measurements also help monitor the patient's response to therapy.

Normal hemoglobin values vary with age and sex. The following ranges serve as a guide:
- Men—14 to 18 g/dl
- Women—12 to 16 g/dl
- Children—11 to 13 g/dl.

A below-normal hemoglobin concentration may result from anemia, recent hemorrhage, or fluid retention, causing hemodilution. An elevated hemoglobin concentration suggests hemoconcentration from polycythemia or dehydration.

Hematocrit. The hematocrit test measures the percentage of red cells in a whole blood sample. Also called the packed red cell volume test, the hematocrit test helps diagnose anemia, polycythemia, and abnormal hydration states. It also helps calculate red cell indices.

Continued on page 19

Normal hematocrit: Age and sex variations

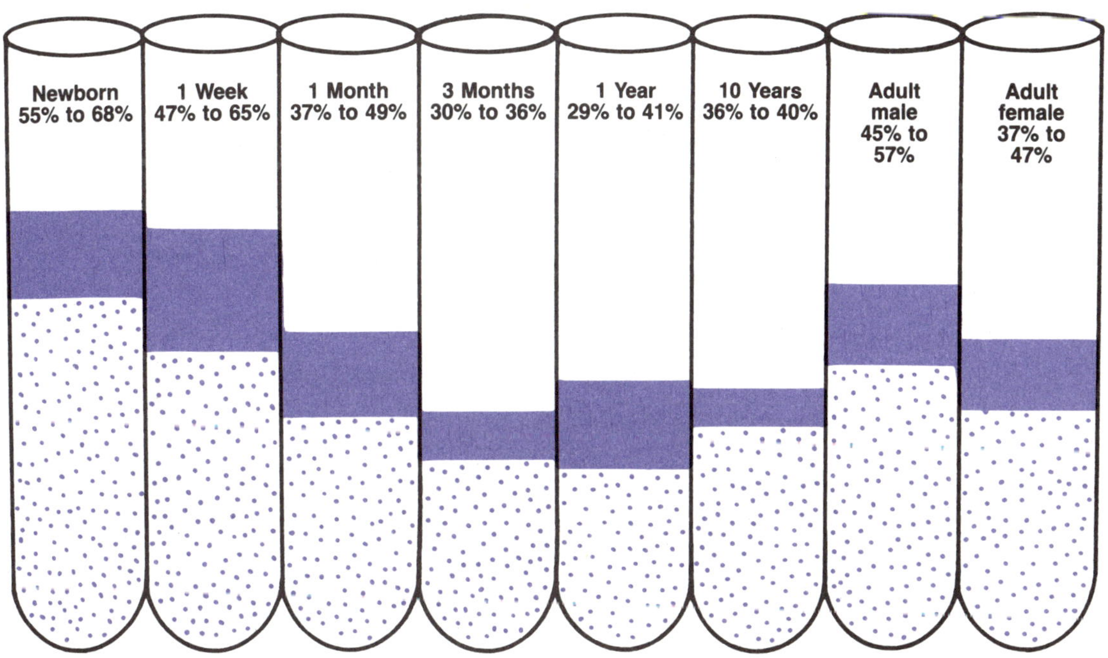

Diagnostic Studies

Red blood cell morphology: Recognizing abnormalities

The normal red blood cell (RBC) has a circular shape with a diameter from 7 μ to to 8 μ and distinct margins. Its center stains less intensely than its periphery. A flexible cell, the RBC contains no nucleus or mitochondria and lives for about 120 days.

Various RBC abnormalities can occur, including shape distortion, fragmentation caused by missing cell membrane pieces, abnormal inclusions, and size variations. The following chart lists RBC abnormalities and the disorders associated with each type.

SHAPE ABNORMALITIES

Cell	Description	Cause	Disorder
Acanthocyte 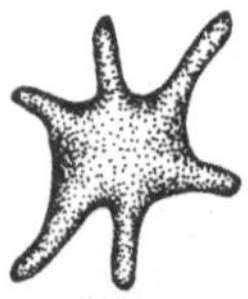	• Normal or slightly reduced in size • Three to twelve blunted needlelike projections of uneven lengths • Saturated with hemoglobin	• Specific physiologic mechanism unknown; excess cholesterol and decreased lecithin appear on RBC membrane	• Congenital abetalipoproteinemia • Hypothyroidism • Severe hepatic disease • Vitamin E deficiency
Target cell 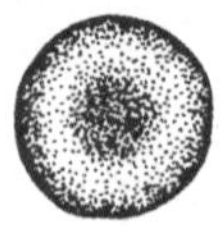	• Bell-shaped when circulating • Target-shaped on smear (dark center and dark outer ring, separated by pale ring)	• Excess cholesterol and phospholipids on RBC membrane	• Hepatic disease • Sickle-cell anemia • Thalassemia
Ovalocyte 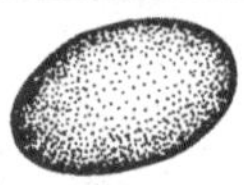	• Egg-shaped • Possibly hypochromic (pale)	• Not well defined	• Iron-deficiency anemia • Myelodysplasia • Sickle-cell anemia • Thalassemia
Sickle cell 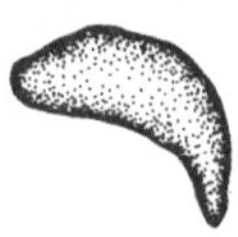	• Sickle-shaped • Rigid, inflexible	• RBC transformed by hemoglobin polymerization stemming from low oxygen tension. Repeated sickling leads to irreversibility.	• Sickle-cell anemia

FRAGMENTATION

Cell	Description	Cause	Disorder
Dacryocyte (Teardrop cell) 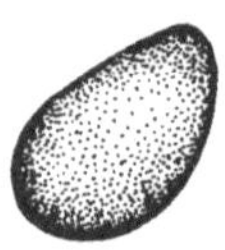	• Teardrop-shaped	• Physiologic mechanism unknown. As cells containing large inclusions try to pass through microcirculation, the portion with inclusion gets pinched off, leaving a tail at end.	• Hypersplenism • Megaloblastic anemia • Thalassemia
Helmet cell 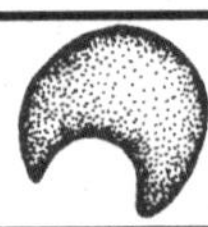	• Helmet-shaped with two projections surrounding empty area	• Abnormal pitting by spleen	• Disseminated intravascular coagulation (DIC) • Myeloid metaplasia • Pulmonary emboli
Keratocyte (burr cell) 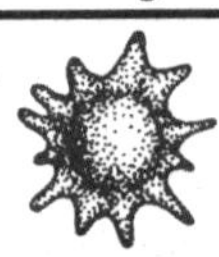	• 10 to 30 projecting spicules • Normochromic • Normocytic	• Intravascular fluid level changes	• Azotemia • Dehydration
Schistocytes 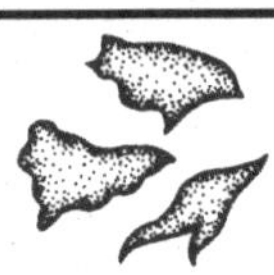	• Bizarrely shaped • Whole pieces missing	• RBC impact with fibrin strands, diseased vessel walls, and artificial surfaces in circulation	• DIC • Microangiopathic hemolytic anemia • Severe burns • Thrombotic thrombocytopenic purpura

ABNORMAL INCLUSIONS

Structure	Description	Cause	Disorder
Basophilic stippling 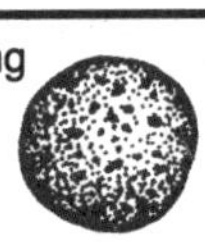	• Fine, coarse, or punctated inclusion	• Precipitated ribonucleoprotein and mitochondrial remnants	• Defective heme synthesis • Metal poisoning • Severe bacterial infection

continued

Diagnostic Studies

Red blood cell morphology: Recognizing abnormalities—*continued*

ABNORMAL INCLUSIONS—*continued*

Structure		Description	Cause	Disorder
Cabot's ring body	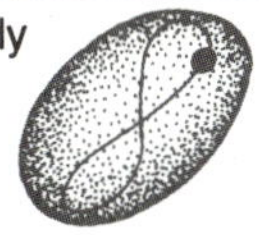	• Inclusions in a figure-eight formation • RBC distorted to look like elongated necklace bead	• Unknown	• Megaloblastic anemia • Postsplenectomy • Thalassemia
Heinz bodies	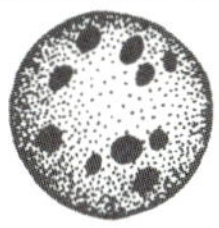	• Large and rigid inclusions that distort cell membrane	• Denatured/precipitated hemoglobin	• G6PD deficiency • Unstable hemoglobin syndromes
Howell-Jolly body	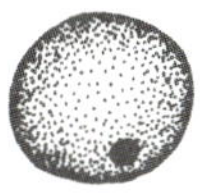	• DNA chromosome piece left in cytoplasm after nucleus departs	• Accelerated or abnormal erythropoiesis triggered by stress (Normally, spleen removes these bodies, but it can't keep up with their formation during stress.)	• Hemolytic anemia • Megaloblastic anemia • Postsplenectomy • Thalassemia
Pappenheimer bodies (siderotic granules)	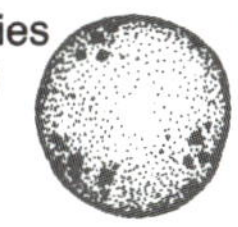	• Small, irregular magenta inclusions that appear in clusters along periphery	• Excess iron stores	• Hemoglobinopathies • Postsplenectomy • Sideroblastic anemia

SIZE VARIATIONS (anisocytosis)

Cell		Description	Cause	Disorder
Macrocytes	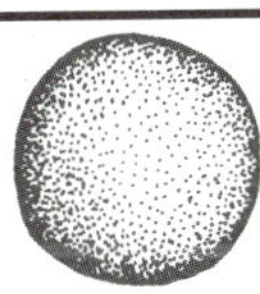	• Greater than 9 μ in diameter	• Impaired DNA synthesis • Chemotherapy	• Hypothyroidism • Megaloblastic anemia • Myelodysplasia
Microcytes	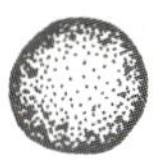	• Less than 7 μ in diameter	• Impaired hemoglobin synthesis	• Anemia of chronic disease • Iron-deficiency anemia • Sideroblastic anemia • Thalassemia

Blood tests—*continued*

Although normal hematocrit varies widely, it amounts to roughly three times the hemoglobin concentration, as indicated below:
- Men—45% to 57%
- Women—37% to 47%
- Children—36% to 40%.

Below-normal hematocrit suggests anemia or hemodilution. Above-normal hematocrit indicates polycythemia or hemoconcentration from blood loss.

With a significant decrease in hematocrit, RBC count, or hemoglobin value, the patient may complain that he feels cold. He may also report these signs and symptoms:
- fatigue
- dyspnea
- tachycardia
- pallor.

These findings occur with different laboratory values in different individuals. The patient may tolerate gradual blood loss, which gives the body time to develop compensatory mechanisms. A massive hemorrhage, on the other hand, produces immediate symptoms.

Continued on page 20

Diagnostic Studies

Anemias: Comparing red cell indices

Red cell indices	Normal values (normocytic, normochromic)	Iron-deficiency anemia (microcytic, hypochromic)	Vitamin B_{12} deficiency anemia (macrocytic, normochromic)
MCV	84 to 99 μ^3	60 to 80 μ^3	95 to 150 μ^3
MCH	26 to 32 pg	5 to 25 pg	33 to 53 pg
MCHC	30% to 36%	20% to 30%	33% to 38%

Blood tests—*continued*

Erythrocyte (RBC) indices. These measure RBC size and hemoglobin content. The indices include mean corpuscular volume (MCV), mean corpuscular hemoglobin (MCH), and mean corpuscular hemoglobin concentration (MCHC).

MCV—the ratio of hematocrit (packed cell volume) to the RBC count—expresses the RBCs' average size and indicates whether they're undersized (microcytic), oversized (macrocytic), or normal (normocytic). MCH—the hemoglobin-RBC ratio—reflects the hemoglobin weight in an average RBC. MCHC—the ratio of hemoglobin weight to hematocrit—measures the hemoglobin concentration in 100 ml of packed red cells. The MCHC value helps distinguish normally colored (normochromic) red cells from paler (hypochromic) red cells.

Normal values for red cell indices include the following:
- MCV—84 to 99 μ^3
- MCH—26 to 32 pg
- MCHC—30% to 36%.

Below-normal MCV and MCHC levels suggest microcytic, hypochromic anemias and thalassemia. A decreased MCH value also appears with microcytic anemia. An increased MCV value indicates macrocytic anemia or folic acid or vitamin B_{12} deficiency anemias. An above-normal MCHC level indicates spherocytosis; an above-normal MCH level, macrocytic anemia.

WBC count. The WBC, or leukocyte, count measures the number of WBCs in a microliter of whole blood. It helps detect infection or inflammation and is useful for monitoring the patient's response to chemotherapy or radiation therapy. Normal values range from 4,100 to 10,900/μl. However, serial WBC counts may vary as much as 2,000, depending on such factors as exercise and stress. Although the count may rise or fall significantly with certain diseases, it proves diagnostically useful only when interpreted in relation to the WBC differential and the patient's clinical status.

A decreased WBC count (leukopenia) indicates bone marrow depression. Possible causes include viral infection or toxic reactions, such as those following antineoplastic treatment; mercury or other heavy metal ingestion; or benzene or arsenic exposure. An elevated WBC count (leukocytosis) may signal infection, leukemia, or tissue necrosis.

WBC differential. This test uses a stained film of peripheal blood to classify 100 or more white cells according to the five major

Diagnostic Studies

types—neutrophils, eosinophils, basophils, lymphocytes, and monocytes—computing the percentage for each. This percentage, or value, constitutes the differential. Multiplying each relative value by the total WBC count yields the absolute number for each white cell type.

The WBC differential, which evaluates the body's capacity to resist and overcome infection, determines an infection's stage and severity and helps detect and identify leukemia types. Remember, for an accurate evaluation, interpret WBC differential values in relation to the total WBC count.

Continued on page 22

How disease affects the white blood cell count

Increased by:	Decreased by:
NEUTROPHILS	
• Infections: osteomyelitis, otitis media, salpingitis, septicemia, gonorrhea, endocarditis, smallpox, chicken pox, herpes, Rocky Mountain spotted fever • Ischemic necrosis from myocardial infarction, burns, carcinoma • Metabolic disorders: diabetic acidosis, eclampsia, uremia, thyrotoxicosis • Stress response from acute hemorrhage, surgery, excessive exercise, emotional distress, third trimester of pregnancy, childbirth • Inflammatory diseases: rheumatic fever, rheumatoid arthritis, acute gout, vasculitis, myositis	• Bone marrow depression from radiation or cytotoxic drugs • Infections: typhoid, tularemia, brucellosis, hepatitis, influenza, measles, mumps, rubella, infectious mononucleosis • Hypersplenism: hepatic disease, storage diseases • Collagen vascular diseases, such as systemic lupus erythematosus • Deficiency of folic acid or vitamin B_{12}
EOSINOPHILS	
• Allergic disorders: asthma, hay fever, food or drug sensitivity, serum sickness, angioneurotic edema • Parasitic infections: trichinosis, hookworm, roundworm, amebiasis • Skin diseases: eczema, pemphigus, psoriasis, dermatitis herpetiformis • Neoplastic diseases: chronic myelocytic leukemia, Hodgkin's disease, metastasis and necrosis of solid tumors • Miscellaneous: collagen vascular diseases, adrenocortical hypofunction, ulcerative colitis, polyarteritis nodosa, postsplenectomy, pernicious anemia, scarlet fever, excessive exercise	• Stress response from trauma, shock, burns, surgery, mental distress • Cushing's syndrome
BASOPHILS	
• Chronic myelocytic leukemia, polycythemia vera, some chronic hemolytic anemias, Hodgkin's disease, systemic mastocytosis, myxedema, ulcerative colitis, chronic hypersensitivity states, nephrosis	• Hyperthyroidism, ovulation, pregnancy, stress
LYMPHOCYTES	
• Infections: pertussis, brucellosis, syphilis, tuberculosis, hepatitis, infectious mononucleosis, mumps, German measles, cytomegalovirus • Other: thyrotoxicosis, hypoadrenalism, ulcerative colitis, immune diseases, lymphocytic leukemia	• Severe debilitating illness, such as congestive heart failure, renal failure, advanced tuberculosis • Defective lymphatic circulation, high levels of adrenal corticosteroids, immunodeficiency from immunosuppressives
MONOCYTES	
• Infections: subacute bacterial endocarditis, tuberculosis, hepatitis, malaria, Rocky Mountain spotted fever • Collagen vascular diseases: systemic lupus erythematosus, rheumatoid arthritis, polyarteritis nodosa • Carcinomas • Monocytic leukemia • Lymphomas	

Diagnostic Studies

Interpreting the WBC differential: Calculating absolute values

For an accurate interpretation of your patient's test results, consider both the relative and absolute differential values of white blood cells (WBCs). Calculate absolute value (number of cells per microliter [μl]) by multiplying the total WBC count by the relative value (a percentage). By themselves, relative values may suggest a particular disorder while masking the true disorder that absolute values reveal. For example, consider a patient with a WBC count of 6,000/μl and a differential showing 30% neutrophils and 50% lymphocytes. His relative lymphocyte count seems above normal (lymphocytosis). However, when multiplied by his WBC count (6,000 × 50% = 3,000 lymphocytes/μl), the absolute lymphocyte count appears well within the normal range.

This same patient also seems to have a below-normal neutrophil count. When multiplied by the WBC count (6,000 × 30% = 1,800 neutrophils/μl), the neutrophil count remains in the below-normal range, indicating that the patient may have a depressed bone marrow.

Selected drugs that affect the eosinophil count

When evaluating your patient's eosinophil count, keep in mind that certain drugs may influence test results. For example, desipramine and methysergide may increase or decrease the eosinophil count; indomethacin or procainamide may decrease it.

The following drugs can increase the eosinophil count by causing an allergic reaction:
- anticonvulsants
- capreomycin
- cephalosporins
- D-penicillamine
- gold compounds
- isoniazid
- nalidixic acid
- para-aminosalicylic acid
- paramomycin
- penicillins
- phenothiazines
- rifampin
- streptomycin
- sulfonamides
- tetracyclines.

Blood tests—*continued*

Here are the normal WBC differential values for white cell types:
- Neutrophils—50% to 60% relative value; 3,000 to 7,000/μl absolute value
- Eosinophils—1% to 4% relative value; 50 to 400/μl absolute value
- Basophils—0.5% to 2.0% relative value; 25 to 100/μl absolute value
- Lymphocytes—20% to 40% relative value; 1,000 to 4,000/μl absolute value
- Monocytes—2% to 9% relative value; 100 to 600/μl absolute value.

Note: Although experts know little about eosinophil function, abnormally high eosinophil levels appear with various allergic reactions and parasitic infections. In patients with these conditions, a separate eosinophil count may prove useful as a follow-up study to the WBC differential. An eosinophil count may also prove appropriate when the WBC differential shows a depressed eosinophil level. (See *Selected drugs that affect the eosinophil count.*)

Platelet count. This test evaluates platelet (thrombocyte) production, which is necessary for blood clotting. Accurate counts prove vital for monitoring chemotherapy and radiation therapy and for assessing the severity of thrombocytosis (abnormally increased platelet count) or thrombocytopenia (abnormally decreased platelet count).

The platelet count normally increases at high temperatures and during strenuous exercise or excitement. The count decreases just before menstruation. *Normal values* vary from 130,000 to 370,000/μl. A platelet count below 50,000/μl can result in spontaneous bleeding; a count below 5,000 usually indicates massive hemorrhage.

A decreased platelet count may result from aplastic or hypoplastic bone marrow, infiltrative bone marrow disease (cancer, leukemia, disseminated infection), megakaryocytic hypoplasia, ineffective thrombopoiesis stemming from folic acid or vitamin B_{12} deficiency, platelet pooling in an enlarged spleen, increased platelet destruction by drugs or immune disorders, disseminated intravascular coagulation (DIC), or mechanical injury to platelets.

An increased platelet count may result from hemorrhage, infectious disorders, cancer, iron-deficiency anemia, surgery, pregnancy, splenectomy, or an inflammatory disorder (for example, a collagen vascular disease). In these cases, the platelet count returns to normal after the primary disorder resolves. However, the platelet count remains high in the patient with primary thrombocytosis, myelofibrosis with myeloid metaplasia, polycythemia vera, or chronic myelocytic leukemia.

An abnormal platelet count usually necessitates further diagnostic studies. These studies may include a CBC, bone marrow biopsy, direct antiglobulin test (direct Coombs' test), and serum protein electrophoresis.

Special RBC tests

Certain RBC tests help monitor cancer and inflammation progress, differentiate anemias, distinguish hemoglobin molecules, and identify antibodies on the patient's RBCs or in his serum. These tests

Diagnostic Studies

include the erythrocyte sedimentation rate, the reticulocyte count, hemoglobin electrophoresis, direct and indirect antiglobulin tests, and RBC survival tests.

Erythrocyte sedimentation rate (ESR). This test measures the rate per time unit (usually 1 hour) at which RBCs in unclotted blood settle to the bottom of a vertical test tube. The faster the cells settle, the higher the ESR.

The settling results from surface changes on the RBCs that cause them to stick together in a column (rouleau formation). These changes stem from plasma alterations (mostly affecting plasma proteins).

The ESR helps monitor the progress of cancer or inflammation. It also helps diagnose occult disease, such as tissue necrosis or connective tissue disease, when other chemical or physical signs appear normal. (Inflammation and necrosis alter the blood proteins that cause RBCs to clump and settle.)

A *normal* ESR varies from 0 to 20 mm/hour. The laboratory method and collection tube type can affect the ESR. Also, the ESR gradually increases with age.

In some diseases, the ESR varies directly with disease severity. A decreased ESR suggests hypofibrinogenemia, sickle-cell anemia, or polycythemia. An elevated ESR may indicate certain cancers, inflammation, infection, cell or tissue necrosis, acute heavy metal poisoning, or severe anemia. However, the ESR may remain normal in many diseases.

Reticulocyte count. This measurement determines the percentage of reticulocytes (immature, nonnucleated RBCs) in the total RBC count. The percentage is expressed as the number of reticulocytes per 1,000 erythrocytes. The reticulocyte count helps assess bone marrow activity. Specifically, this test can:

- distinguish between anemias resulting from bone marrow failure and those resulting from RBC destruction, which may occur with hemorrhage or hemolysis

Continued on page 24

Erythrocyte sedimentation rate test: An aid to disease differentiation

Although not useful for primary diagnosis, the erythrocyte sedimentation rate (ESR) test may help differentiate among diseases with similar signs and symptoms (grouped together in the table below).

Possible underlying disease	ESR result
Bacterial infection Viral infection	• Above normal • Normal
Acute appendicitis Acute pelvic inflammatory disease, ectopic pregnancy	• Normal • Above normal
Acute myocardial infarction Angina pectoris	• Above normal • Normal
Osteoarthritis Rheumatic fever Rheumatoid arthritis	• Normal • Above normal • Above normal

Diagnostic Studies

Blood tests—*continued*

- monitor therapy for vitamin B_{12} deficiency anemia
- assess bone marrow recovery in aplastic anemia
- measure the effects of radiation on exposed workers.

The following ranges show normal reticulocyte count values:
- Men—0.5% to 1.5%
- Women—0.5% to 2.5%
- Children—0.5% to 4%.

A low reticulocyte count (reticulocytopenia) signals decreased RBC production by the bone marrow. This condition may indicate aplastic anemia, iron-deficiency anemia, vitamin B_{12} deficiency anemia, chronic infection, or radiation therapy.

A high count (reticulocytosis) suggests accelerated RBC production as the bone marrow replaces lost or destroyed cells. A patient with a high count may have hemolytic anemia, sickle-cell anemia, metastatic cancer, leukemia, or hereditary spherocytosis. A high count may also appear after a splenectomy or 3 or 4 days after hemorrhage. An increase may also indicate treatment effectiveness for anemia. For example, a patient receiving iron therapy for iron-deficiency anemia may show more than a 20% reticulocyte count increase. Transfusion for vitamin B_{12} deficiency anemia also causes the reticulocyte count to rise.

Hemoglobin electrophoresis. This procedure uses an electric field to separate hemoglobin molecules, which move through the field at different speeds based on their electrical charge. They create distinctive pigmented bands used for comparison with known standards for different hemoglobins.

Hemoglobin electrophoresis detects normal and abnormal hemoglobins, which is useful in diagnosing such hemolytic diseases as thalassemias. (For more information on abnormal hemoglobins, see *Hemoglobin type and distribution: Recognizing variations.*)

Normally, the hemoglobin A molecule is the most common form in adults, accounting for over 95% of the total hemoglobin. Hemoglo-

Hemoglobin type and distribution: Recognizing variations

Hemoglobin (Hgb)	Percentage of total hemoglobin	Clinical implications
Hgb A_2	4% to 5.8% Under 2%	• β-thalassemia minor • Hgb H disease
Hgb F (in adults)	2% to 5% 10% to 90% 5% to 15% 5% to 35% 100% 15%	• β-thalassemia minor • β-thalassemia major • β-δ-thalassemia minor • Heterozygous hereditary persistence of fetal hemoglobin (HPFH) • Homozygous HPFH • Homozygous Hgb S
Homozygous Hgb S	70% to 98%	• Sickle-cell disease
Homozygous Hgb C	90% to 98%	• Hgb C disease
Heterozygous Hgb C	24% to 44%	• Hemoglobin C trait

Diagnostic Studies

bins A_2 and F (fetal hemoglobins) normally appear only in minute quantities—about 2% to 3% for hemoglobin A_2 and less than 1% for hemoglobin F. In newborns, hemoglobin F constitutes half the total hemoglobin.

Amino acid variations in hemoglobin's globin portion create more than 350 abnormal variants. Because these variants usually produce no symptoms, they remain clinically unimportant. The best known abnormal variants include hemoglobin S (responsible for sickle-cell anemia) and hemoglobin C (which causes mild hemolytic anemia). The most common abnormality involves a significant hemoglobin A_2 increase. Diagnostic for thalassemia minor, this abnormality may cause a mild anemia but usually produces no symptoms.

Note: Researchers initially identified hemoglobin variants by letter but now name them after the place where they discovered them, such as Philadelphia (G-Philadelphia), Ann Arbor, Dakar, and Hiroshima.

Direct and indirect antiglobulin tests. These tests use antigen-antibody reactions to help diagnose various hematologic disorders and to identify minor blood groups, such as the Kell blood group system. The direct antiglobulin test (DAGT), also known as the direct Coombs' test, reveals antibodies on the patient's RBCs. The indirect antiglobulin test (IAGT), or indirect Coombs' test, detects antibodies in the serum.

A negative result is normal for the DAGT and the IAGT. A positive DAGT suggests autoimmune hemolytic anemia (in which the body produces antibodies that coat its blood cells), transfusion reaction (in which incompatible blood sensitizes the patient's blood cells), erythroblastosis fetalis (in which maternal antibodies sensitize fetal RBCs), or drug-induced RBC sensitization.

A specific antibody, usually arising from a previous transfusion or pregnancy (Rh-negative factor), produces a positive IAGT result. A nonspecific antibody, which may arise in such conditions as cold agglutination disease or drug-induced hemolytic anemia, also produces a positive IAGT result.

RBC survival tests. These studies include the osmotic fragility (erythrocyte fragility) test and the RBC survival time test.

The *osmotic fragility test* relies on osmosis—fluid movement across a membrane from a less concentrated solution to a more concentrated one. Using this natural tendency to correct the imbalance, this test can confirm RBC morphologic abnormalities. It measures erythrocyte resistance to hemolysis in increasingly dilute saline solutions, usually ranging from 0.7% to 0.3%. In each solution, fluid enters the cell, causing it to swell. Eventually, the cell can hold no more water and then bursts. The closer the saline concentration comes to that of normal plasma (0.85 g/dl) when hemolysis occurs, the more fragile the cell. Normal erythrocytes begin to lyse in 0.45% to 0.39% saline solutions.

Below-normal cell fragility suggests sickle-cell anemia, iron-deficiency anemia, polycythemia vera, or thalassemia. Above-normal

Continued on page 26

Diagnostic Studies

Blood tests—*continued*

cell fragility may occur with hemolytic anemia, chemical poisons, burns, or autoimmune hemolytic anemia.

The *RBC survival time test* measures the survival time of circulating RBCs and detects abnormal RBC sequestration and destruction sites, using a radioactive label to trace RBCs in the body. Normally, RBC destruction occurs only when cells are senescent. However, in hemolytic disorders, destruction occurs in RBCs of all ages.

The test mixes a sample of the patient's own RBCs with radioactive chromium-51 sodium chromate (^{51}Cr). The ^{51}Cr crosses RBC membranes and reduces to chromium ion, which binds to hemoglobin. The labeled RBCs are then injected into the patient's bloodstream. Over the next 3 to 4 weeks, serial blood samples measure the percentage of labeled cells in a unit volume. The test ends when half the labeled cells disappear, corresponding to random destruction.

During the test period, a gamma camera scans the body for areas with abnormally high radiation. These areas indicate sequestration and destruction of the labeled cells, thus releasing radioactively labeled hemoglobin. The gamma scan helps direct treatment. For example, if it detects excessive radiation in the spleen, the doctor may recommend a splenectomy.

The normal half-life of erythrocytes labeled with ^{51}Cr ranges from 25 to 35 days. (*Note:* A normal RBC survives about 120 days [it has a half-life of 60 days]. ^{51}Cr-labeled RBCs have a shorter half-life because about 1% of senescent RBCs leave the circulation each day and about 1% of the ^{51}Cr spontaneously escapes from labeled RBCs each day.)

Normal gamma scans may show slight radioactivity in the spleen, the liver, and the bone marrow. Half the plasma radioactivity disappears after 1 or 2 hours. In the stool, radioactively labeled hemoglobin should amount to less than 3 ml in 24 hours.

Decreased RBC survival time suggests a hemolytic disease, such as chronic lymphocytic leukemia, congenital nonspherocytic hemolytic anemia, hemoglobin C disease, hereditary spherocytosis, idiopathic acquired hemolytic anemia, paroxysmal nocturnal hemoglobinuria, elliptocytosis, vitamin B_{12} deficiency anemia, sickle-cell anemia, sickle-cell hemoglobin C disease, or hemolytic-uremic syndrome.

Along with the RBC survival time test, the doctor may order stool checks to detect GI bleeding; hematocrit test; blood volume studies; and radionuclide iron uptake and clearance tests to help determine the specific anemia present.

An actively bleeding patient shouldn't undergo the RBC survival time test. Nor should a patient receive blood transfusions during the test period. As the test progresses, be sure to record and report signs of active bleeding immediately.

Diagnostic Studies

Coagulation studies: Ensuring accuracy

Follow these guidelines to ensure the most accurate coagulation test results:
- Perform a clean venipuncture—blood contaminated with tissue thromboplastin will cause misleading test results.
- Use plastic syringes when drawing a blood sample to test for Factors XI and XII.
- Allow no more than 4 hours between blood sampling and coagulation testing. Allow only 2 hours between blood centrifugation and coagulation testing because, once centrifuged, red blood cells lose their buffering effect on the plasma.
- Place the blood sample on ice immediately after sampling, to preserve its labile factors.
- Avoid using hemolyzed plasma, which may yield decreased clotting times.

Coagulation screening tests

These studies help detect bleeding disorders and specific coagulation defects (see *Coagulation studies: Ensuring accuracy*). We'll discuss these common tests:
- bleeding time
- capillary fragility
- activated partial thromboplastin time
- prothrombin time
- plasma thrombin time
- fibrin split products.

(For details on platelet count, see the section "Complete blood count (CBC)," page 16.)

Bleeding time. This test measures the body's ability to stop bleeding after a standard skin incision. Bleeding time depends on blood vessel wall elasticity, platelet numbers, and ability to form the hemostatic plug. Likely candidates for the bleeding time test include patients with a personal or family history indicating bleeding abnormalities. Along with a platelet count, this test also helps screen patients scheduled for surgery.

The bleeding time test proves especially useful in detecting vascular abnormalities and can help detect platelet abnormalities or deficiencies. Although the test may also help detect thrombocytopenia, a stained RBC examination and platelet count are far more effective. The bleeding time test has little value in identifying individuals at risk for bleeding from aspirin use. It's not recommended for a patient whose platelet count is less than 75,000/μl. However, some patients with altered platelet morphology can have normal bleeding times despite low platelet counts.

Four methods can measure bleeding time: Duke, Ivy, template, and modified template. Used most often, the template methods prove most accurate because they standardize the incision size, making test results reproducible. Normal bleeding times for the four test methods are the following:
- Duke method—1 to 3 minutes
- Ivy method—1 to 7 minutes
- template method—2 to 8 minutes
- modified template method—2 to 10 minutes.

Prolonged bleeding time occurs with several disorders associated with thrombocytopenia, including Hodgkin's disease, acute leukemia, DIC, newborn hemolytic disease, Schönlein-Henoch purpura, severe hepatic disease (such as cirrhosis), and severe deficiency of Factors I, II, V, VII, VIII, IX, or XI. Prolonged bleeding time with a normal platelet count indicates a platelet function disorder, such as thrombasthenia or thrombocytopathia. Either of these abnormal test results warrants follow-up clot retraction, prothrombin consumption, and platelet aggregation tests.

Remember, a single prolonged bleeding time result doesn't verify hemorrhagic disease; such a result may stem from the cutting of a large vessel, which lengthens the time needed for bleeding to stop. To guard against this possibility, the test should include two punctures and the test results should be averaged.

Continued on page 28

Diagnostic Studies

Positive capillary fragility test

Hemorrhagic disorders, such as thrombocytopenia, produce a strong showing of petechiae below the application site of the blood pressure cuff. The appearance of a number of petechiae indicates abnormality.

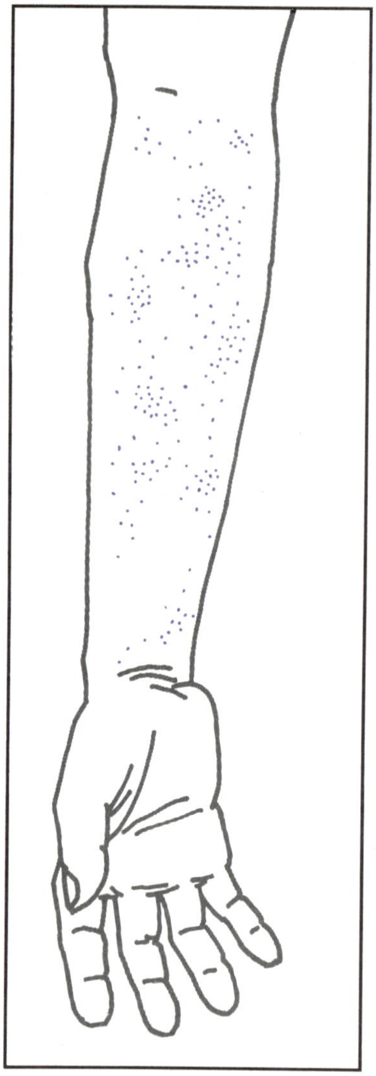

Blood tests—*continued*

guard against this possibility, the test should include two punctures and the test results should be averaged.

Capillary fragility test. Also known as the tourniquet test, positive-pressure test, or Rumpel-Leede capillary fragility test, this study measures the capillaries' ability to remain intact under increasing intracapillary pressure.

For this test, a blood pressure cuff is wrapped around the patient's upper arm and the blood pressure increased to a level midway between the systolic and diastolic blood pressures, but no higher than 100 mm Hg. At this pressure, blood can enter the arm and hand but can't return to circulation easily. The pressure, which must remain elevated for 5 minutes, may cause capillary bleeding indicated by petechiae on the arm, wrist, or hand. The number of petechiae in a given circular space constitutes the test result.

Some petechiae may appear even before the test. Fewer than 10 petechiae on the forearm 5 minutes after the test reflects a normal, or negative, result; more than 10 reflects a positive result. You can use the following scale to report test results:
- 0 to 10 petechiae = 1+
- 11 to 20 petechiae = 2+
- 21 to 50 petechiae = 3+
- 51 or more petechiae = 4+.

A positive finding indicates capillary wall weakness (vascular purpura) or a platelet defect. It occurs in such conditions as thrombocytopenia, thrombasthenia, purpura senilis, scurvy, DIC, von Willebrand's disease, vitamin K deficiency, dysproteinemia, polycythemia vera, and severe deficiencies of Factor VII, fibrinogen, or prothrombin. Capillary fragility may also increase in conditions unrelated to bleeding defects, including scarlet fever, measles, influenza, chronic renal disease, hypertension, and diabetes with coexistent vascular disease. A positive test sometimes appears before menstruation and at other times in some healthy individuals, especially in women over age 40.

Activated partial thromboplastin time (APTT). The APTT test evaluates all intrinsic pathway clotting factors (except Factors VII and XIII) by measuring the time needed for a fibrin clot to form after the addition of calcium and phospholipid emulsion to a plasma sample. The APTT relies on the activator kaolin to shorten clotting time. (*Note:* The partial thromboplastin time, a similar test, is less sensitive and less commonly performed.)

Because most congenital coagulation deficiencies (described in Chapter 5) occur in the intrinsic pathway, the APTT test proves valuable in preoperative screening for bleeding tendencies. It also serves as the preferred test for monitoring heparin therapy.

Normally, a fibrin clot forms 25 to 36 seconds after reagent addition. Prolonged times may mean that the plasma sample contains:
- plasma clotting factor deficiencies
- heparin
- fibrin split products or fibrinolysins
- circulating anticoagulants that act as antibodies to clotting factors.

Diagnostic Studies

Prothrombin time (PT). This test measures the time required for a fibrin clot to form in a citrated plasma sample after the addition of calcium ion and tissue thromboplastin (Factor III). It then compares this time with the fibrin clotting time in a plasma control sample.

The PT test reaction bypasses the intrinsic coagulation pathway (plasma thromboplastin formation in Stage I) and doesn't involve platelets. Therefore, it indirectly measures prothrombin and serves as an excellent screening method for evaluating prothrombin, fibrinogen, and extrinsic coagulation Factors V, VII, and X. It's the preferred test for monitoring oral anticoagulant therapy.

Test results commonly appear as percentages of normal activity compared with a curve of the clotting rate of normal diluted plasma. However, this method's inaccurate because sample dilution affects the coagulation mechanism. A more accurate reporting method provides both the patient's and the control's clotting times in seconds.

Normal PT values vary with sex. In men, they range from 9.6 to 11.8 seconds; in women, from 9.5 to 11.3 seconds. Values also vary with the tissue thromboplastin source and the sensing device that measures clot formation. In a patient receiving oral anticoagulants, PT usually remains between one and a half and two times the normal control value.

A prolonged PT may mean a deficiency in fibrinogen, prothrombin, or Factors V, VII, or X. (Specific tests can pinpoint the deficient factor.) Vitamin K deficiency or hepatic disease can also prolong PT, as can ongoing oral anticoagulant therapy. A PT that exceeds two and a half times the control value commonly appears with abnormal bleeding.

Plasma thrombin time. This test, also known as the thrombin clotting time test, measures how quickly a clot forms after the addition of a standard amount of bovine thrombin to a platelet-poor plasma sample from the patient and to a normal plasma control sample. Because thrombin rapidly converts fibrinogen to a fibrin clot, this procedure provides a quick, although imprecise, estimate of plasma fibrinogen levels.

The plasma thrombin time test helps detect a fibrinogen deficiency or defect, diagnose DIC and hepatic disease, and monitor heparin, streptokinase, or urokinase therapy.

Normal plasma thrombin times range from 10 to 15 seconds. Reported test results usually include control values. A plasma thrombin time greater than 1.3 times the control may mean effective heparin therapy, hepatic disease, DIC, hypofibrinogenemia, or dysfibrinogenemia.

A patient with a prolonged plasma thrombin time requires quantitation of fibrinogen levels. If the doctor suspects DIC, he'll also order the fibrin split products test (see below).

Fibrin split products (FSP) test. After a fibrin clot forms in response to vascular injury, the fibrinolytic system acts to prevent excessive

Continued on page 30

Diagnostic Studies

Blood tests—*continued*

clotting. To do so, it converts plasminogen into the fibrin-dissolving enzyme plasmin, which degrades fibrin and fibrinogen into fragments (split products, also called fibrinogen degradation products). Labeled X, Y, D, and E, according to decreasing molecular weight, these fragments may retain some anticoagulant activity. Too many split products in circulation leads to abnormally active fibrinolysis and such coagulation disorders as DIC.

An immunoprecipitation reaction detects FSP. The FSP test uses the serum left in a blood sample after clotting. The test involves mixing the serum on a slide with latex particles carrying D and E split products. These products adhere in clumps if the serum contains fibrin or FSP.

The FSP test helps detect split products in the circulation and diagnose DIC, distinguishing it from other coagulation disorders. It can also determine how much fibrinolysis occurs during coagulation.

In a screening assay, serum normally contains less than 10 mcg/ml of FSP. In a quantitative assay, normal levels fall below 3 mcg/ml.

In primary fibrinolytic states, FSP levels rise from increased circulating profibrinolysin. In secondary states, they rise from DIC and subsequent fibrinolysis. Elevated levels also occur in conditions unrelated to hematologic defects—acute leukemia, alcoholic cirrhosis, postcesarean birth, preeclampsia, abruptio placentae, congenital heart disease, sunstroke, burns, intrauterine death, pulmonary embolus, deep-vein thrombosis (transient increase), and myocardial infarction (after 1 or 2 days). FSP levels usually exceed 100 mcg/ml in active renal disease or renal transplant rejection.

Radiologic studies

These studies help diagnose and stage lymphomas, identify metastatic lymph node involvement, and differentiate primary and secondary lymphedema. They also help evaluate the effectiveness of chemotherapy and radiation therapy. (*Note:* Make sure the patient or a responsible family member signs a consent form before undergoing an invasive radiologic procedure.)

Computed tomography (CT) scan
This advanced imaging technique uses a computer and X-ray absorption to depict subtle differences in tissue density, allowing the doctor to distinguish tumors from cysts. A CT scan also helps stage lymphomas and guide such interventions as needle biopsy and abscess drainage.

The technique produces cross-sectional images (slices) that provide a three-dimensional view of specific body areas when projected sequentially onto a video screen. The scanning machine includes a large ring through which the patient passes on a mechanically sliding table. Pencil-thin X-ray beams pass into the receptor on the side opposite the ring. After 10 to 30 slices, the computer assembles an image.

Diagnostic Studies

A contrast medium can help maximize visible differences in tissue density. The patient undergoing an abdominal CT scan may need to drink a contrast medium, such as flavored low-density barium or Gastrografin, since unopacified bowel regions may simulate abdominal masses. Bowel preparation's unnecessary unless the patient must undergo other barium studies later that same day. For an upper abdominal series, the patient will probably need to drink 300 ml of barium 15 minutes before the films are taken. For a midabdominal or pelvic series, the patient takes 600 ml of barium about 1 hour beforehand, then an additional 300 ml 45 minutes later. For best results, the patient should fast at least 2 hours before taking the barium.

An I.V. contrast medium helps examine a mass for vascular characteristics, differentiate between vascular anomalies and cancerous tumors, opacify the urinary tract, and improve anatomic definition. It can, for example, help determine common bile duct patency.

The patient will receive an I.V. contrast medium by direct I.V. bolus or infusion. A large-gauge needle (18G to 19G) is usually inserted in a medially directed antecubital vein.

Nursing considerations. When preparing your patient for a CT scan, be sure to describe the procedure to him and answer any questions he may have. Tell him that the test should take about 30 to 60 minutes, although he should allow extra time for delays and repeat scans. Instruct him to lie still while the table passes through the ring and to hold his breath when requested. Warn him that he may experience a dye reaction—a hot, flushed sensation; nausea; or a metallic taste in his mouth.

Ask the patient if he's allergic to iodine or shellfish; if he is, notify the radiology department. Tell the patient to report any abnormal reactions he experiences during the procedures. Such reactions may involve the respiratory tract (nasal congestion from mucosal edema, dyspnea from laryngeal edema, stridor, bronchospasms, wheezing, cough, substernal distress, or crackles), the cardiovascular system (syncope from hypotension), and the skin (pruritus of the face, palms, and soles and angioedema from increased vascular permeability). Remember that elderly patients and those with diabetes, compromised renal function, or cardiovascular disease have an increased risk for an adverse reaction to contrast medium.

After the procedure, allow the patient to eat or drink. If he has taken barium, give him a laxative. Observe him for delayed hypersensitivity reactions, especially if he's in any high-risk group mentioned above.

Gallium scan
This total body scan usually takes place 24 to 48 hours after an I.V. radioactive gallium (^{67}Ga) citrate injection. Occasionally, it's performed 72 hours after the injection or, in acute inflammatory disease, 4 to 6 hours afterward.

Although the liver, spleen, bones, and large bowel normally take up gallium, certain benign and cancerous tumors and inflammatory

Continued on page 32

Diagnostic Studies

Radiologic studies—*continued*

lesions also attract the substance. However, many tumors and some inflammatory lesions may not show abnormal gallium activity. Consequently, expect the doctor to order additional tests, such as ultrasonography and a CT scan, to verify the diagnosis.

Gallium scanning proves useful when the site of disease (usually cancer) isn't clearly defined and when the patient's condition won't worsen during the delay between the gallium injection and the scan.

Normal gallium activity appears in the liver, spleen, bones, and large bowel. Abnormal gallium activity may appear with various sarcomas; Wilms' tumor; neuroblastomas; kidney, uterine, vaginal, and stomach cancers; and testicular tumors, including seminoma, embryonal carcinoma, choriocarcinoma, and teratocarcinoma, which commonly metastasize via the lymphatic system.

In Hodgkin's disease and non-Hodgkin's lymphoma, gallium scanning can show abnormal activity in one or more lymph nodes or in extranodal locations. Gallium scanning supported by lymphangiography results can gauge metastatic extent more accurately than either test alone, since neither test consistently identifies all cancerous nodes.

After chemotherapy or radiation therapy, gallium scanning can help detect new or recurrent tumors. However, these therapies can diminish tumor affinity for gallium without eliminating the tumor.

Nursing considerations. When preparing your patient for the procedure, explain the test's purpose and the time required (up to a 48-hour wait after injection, then 30 to 60 minutes for the actual scan). Tell him who will perform the test and where. Inform him that he doesn't need to restrict food or fluids. Administer a laxative and/or cleansing enema, as ordered. Warn him that he may experience transient discomfort from needle puncture during ^{67}Ga injection. Reassure him that the gallium—only slightly radioactive—won't harm him.

In procedures using a gamma scintillation camera, explain that, although the uptake probe and detector head may touch the patient's skin, he won't experience discomfort. If the procedure uses a rectilinear scanner, mention that the machine makes a soft, irregular clicking noise as it registers the radiation emissions.

After the test, administer routine postprocedure care.

Lymphangiography
Also known as lymphography, this test radiographically examines the lymphatic system after injection of an oil-based contrast medium into a lymphatic vessel in each foot or, less commonly, in each hand. Injection into the foot allows visualization of the lymphatics in the leg, the inguinal and iliac regions, and the retroperitoneum up to the thoracic duct. Injection into the hand allows visualization of the axillary and supraclavicular nodes. Less commonly, this procedure can also assess the cervical (retroauricular) region. However, the method's less useful there.

Diagnostic Studies

X-ray films taken immediately after injection show lymphatic system filling. Those taken 24 hours later show the lymph nodes. Because the contrast medium remains in the nodes for up to 2 years, subsequent X-ray films can assess disease progression and monitor treatment effectiveness.

The lymphatic system normally demonstrates homogeneous and complete filling with contrast medium on initial films. On 24-hour films, lymph nodes normally appear fully opacified and well circumscribed. Lymphatic channels should empty a few hours after contrast medium injection.

Enlarged, foamy-looking nodes indicate lymphoma—either Hodgkin's or non-Hodgkin's. Filling defects or failure to opacify indicates metastatic lymph node involvement. The number of nodes affected, any unilateral or bilateral involvement, and the extent of extranodal involvement help determine lymphoma staging. However, definitive staging may require additional diagnostic tests, such as a CT scan and other tomography, ultrasonography, selective biopsy, and laparotomy.

Shortened lymphatic vessels and fewer than normal vessels indicate primary lymphedema. Abruptly terminating lymphatic vessels, resulting from a retroperitoneal tumor impinging on the vessels; inflammation; filariasis; and trauma from surgery or irradiation indicate secondary lymphedema.

Lymphangiography can also help suggest surgical treatment and evaluate the effectiveness of chemotherapy or radiation therapy. A patient with enlarged lymph nodes, detected by CT scan or ultrasonography, may also undergo lymphangiography for more definite diagnosis.

Nursing considerations. To prepare your patient, explain the procedure to him and answer any questions. Inform him that he can eat and drink before the test. Tell him who will perform the procedure and that it takes about 3 hours. Mention that he'll need to return on the following day so that additional films can be taken but that these take less than 30 minutes.

Explain that he'll receive an injection of Ethiodol (ethiodized oil, a 37% iodine–based, blue contrast medium) in each foot to outline lymphatic vessels. Warn him that the injections cause transient discomfort and that the contrast medium will discolor his urine and stool and may tinge his vision blue for 48 hours. His skin may also show a blue tinge, possibly for several months.

Tell him that the doctor will administer a local anesthetic, then make a small incision in each foot and inject the contrast medium through a cannula inserted into a lymphatic vessel. Advise the patient that he must remain as still as possible during the injection, which takes about 1½ hours, and that he may experience some discomfort in the popliteal or inguinal areas when injection begins. If he'll undergo the test as an outpatient, advise him to have a family member or friend accompany him in case he needs support to return home. Warn him that the incision site may feel sore for several days afterward.

Continued on page 34

Diagnostic Studies

Radiologic studies—*continued*

Check the patient's history for a hypersensitivity to iodine, seafood, or the contrast media used in other diagnostic tests, such as CT scans.

Just before the procedure, instruct the patient to urinate; then record his vital signs as a baseline for later comparison. If ordered, administer a sedative and an oral antihistamine (if the doctor suspects a hypersensitivity to the contrast medium).

After inpatient lymphangiography, check the patient's vital signs every 4 hours for 48 hours. Watch for pulmonary complications, such as shortness of breath, pleuritic pain, hypotension, low-grade fever, and cyanosis. These complications indicate embolization of the contrast medium. Enforce bed rest for 24 hours, keeping the patient's feet elevated to reduce swelling, as ordered. Apply ice packs to the incision sites to help reduce swelling, and administer an analgesic, as ordered. Check the incision sites for infection and leave dressings in place for 2 days, making sure the wounds remain dry. Advise the patient that his sutures must stay in place for 7 to 10 days. Give the outpatient and his family similar instructions. Tell them to call the doctor immediately if complications develop.

Other diagnostic tests

The patient with a hematologic problem may also require lymph node biopsy and bone marrow aspiration and needle biopsy.

Lymph node biopsy
This procedure involves either surgical excision of an active lymph node or needle aspiration of a nodal specimen for histologic examination. Both techniques usually involve a local anesthetic and sample superficial nodes in the cervical, supraclavicular, axillary, or inguinal region. Excision, the preferred technique, provides a larger specimen. CBC, liver function studies, liver and spleen scans, and X-rays should precede the biopsy.

During infection, lymph nodes swell from their usual flat bean shape, then return to normal as the infection resolves. The doctor may order lymph node biopsy if nodal enlargement—accompanied by backache, leg edema, breathing and swallowing difficulties, and later weight loss, weakness, severe itching, fever, night sweats, cough, hemoptysis, or hoarseness—persists.

Histologic examination of the biopsy specimen can determine if lymph node enlargement reflects cancerous or noncancerous causes of lymph node enlargement; it can also distinguish between benign and cancerous lymph node tumors. Lymph node biopsy can also stage metastatic lymph node cancer.

Nursing considerations. In preparing your patient for biopsy, describe the procedure and answer any questions. Explain that this test provides lymph node tissue for microscopic study. Also check the patient history for a hypersensitivity to the anesthetic. For excisional biopsy, instruct the patient not to eat after midnight and to drink only clear liquids on the morning of the test. For deeper node biopsy with general anesthesia, he must also restrict fluids. For needle biopsy, inform him that he needn't restrict food or fluids.

Diagnostic Studies

Tell him who will perform the biopsy and where; that the procedure takes 15 to 30 minutes; and that analysis takes a day to complete.

If the patient will receive a local anesthetic, explain that he may experience discomfort during injection. Just before the biopsy, record baseline vital signs.

After the procedure, check your patient's vital signs and monitor for bleeding, tenderness, and redness at the biopsy site. Tell the patient he may resume his normal diet.

Bone marrow aspiration and needle biopsy
Because most hematopoiesis occurs in bone marrow, histologic and hematologic bone marrow examination yields valuable diagnostic information about blood disorders. Bone marrow aspiration and needle biopsy provide the material for that examination.

Aspiration biopsy removes a fluid specimen containing bone marrow cells in suspension. Needle biopsy removes a marrow core containing cells, not fluid. Using both methods provides the best possible marrow specimens.

Bleeding and infection may result from bone marrow biopsy at any site, but the most serious complications occur at the sternum. These complications, although rare, include puncture of the heart and major blood vessels, which causes severe hemorrhage, and puncture of the mediastinum, which causes mediastinitis or pneumomediastinum. (See *Bone marrow aspiration and biopsy sites,* page 36.)

Bone marrow may be red or yellow. Red marrow, which accounts for about 50% of an adult's marrow, contains hematopoietic cells, fat cells, and connective tissue. It actively produces blood cells. The inactive yellow marrow contains fat cells and connective tissue. (Yellow marrow can become active in response to the body's needs, giving the normal adult a large hematopoietic capacity.) An infant's marrow is mainly red.

Bone marrow biopsy helps diagnose thrombocytopenia, leukemias, granulomas, and aplastic, hypoplastic, and vitamin B_{12} deficiency anemias. It also helps evaluate primary and metastatic tumors, determine infection causes, stage such diseases as Hodgkin's disease, evaluate chemotherapy effectiveness, and monitor myelosuppression.

Specifically, histologic examination can help detect myelofibrosis, granulomas, lymphoma, or cancer. Hematologic analysis, including the WBC differential and the myeloid-erythroid ratio, can suggest various disorders.

Also, special stains that detect hematologic disorders produce these normal findings when used on bone marrow:
- +2 level with the iron stain, which measures hemosiderin (storage iron)
- negative with the Sudan Black B (SBB) stain, which shows granulocytes
- negative with the periodic acid-Schiff (PAS) stain, which detects glycogen reactions.

Continued on page 37

Bone marrow biopsy: Preparing a child

If you're caring for a pediatric patient who's scheduled for a bone marrow biopsy, you'll need to take special steps to reduce his anxiety and promote his cooperation. Give him his own biopsy kit containing a syringe (without a needle), cotton balls, and adhesive bandages. Use a doll or stuffed animal to demonstrate the procedure. Answer any questions he may have and be sure to describe the kinds of pressure and discomfort he'll feel during the procedure. That way, you'll gain his confidence.

Before the biopsy, discuss the equipment on the tray. Ask the parents to get involved. They can help you hold the child still and reassure him. Tell the child he'll feel some pain when the doctor removes the bone marrow but that the pain will go away quickly. Let him know that it's OK to cry or yell if he wants to.

Diagnostic Studies

Bone marrow aspiration and biopsy sites

Posterior superior iliac crest is the preferred site, since no vital organs or vessels are located nearby. With the patient in a lateral position with one leg flexed, the doctor inserts the needle several centimeters lateral to the iliosacral junction, entering the bone plane crest with the needle directed downward and toward the anterior inferior spine or entering a few centimeters below the crest at a right angle to the surface of the bone.

Spinous process is preferred if multiple punctures are necessary or if marrow is absent at other sites. In this procedure, the patient sits on the edge of the bed, leaning over the bedside stand; or, if the patient is uncooperative, he may be placed in the prone position with restraints. The doctor selects the spinous process of the third or fourth lumbar vertebrae and inserts the needle at the crest or slightly to one side, advancing the needle in the direction of the bone plane.

Tibia is the site of choice for infants younger than age 1. The infant is placed in a prone position on a bed or an examining table with a sandbag beneath the leg. The foot is taped to the surface of the table, or an assistant holds the leg stationary by placing a hand under it. The doctor inserts the needle about ⅜″ (1 cm) below the tibial tuberosity and slightly toward the medial side, being careful to angle the needle point toward the foot to avoid epiphyseal injury.

Sternum involves the greatest risks and is seldom used for marrow aspiration. For this procedure, the patient is supine on a firm bed or an examining table with a small pillow beneath the shoulders to elevate the chest and lower the head. The doctor secures the needle guard 3 to 4 mm from the tip of the needle to avoid accidental puncture of the heart or a major vessel. Then, he inserts the needle at the midline of the sternum at the second intercostal space.

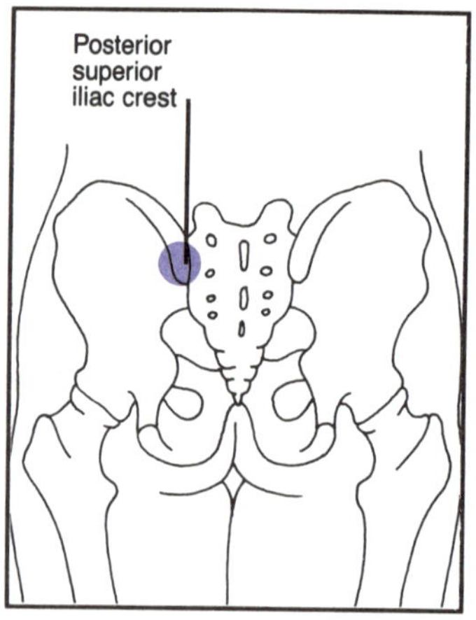

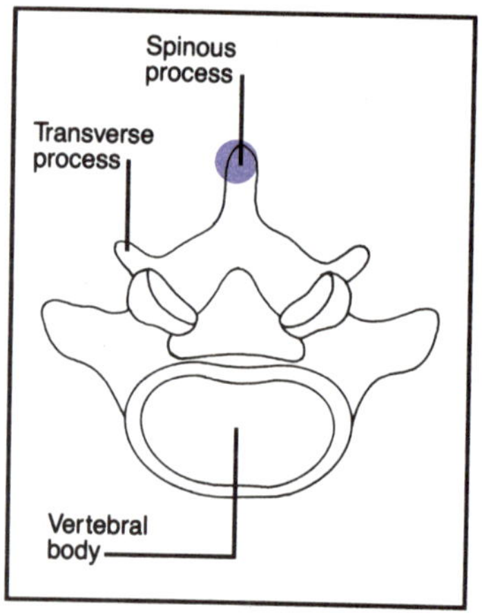

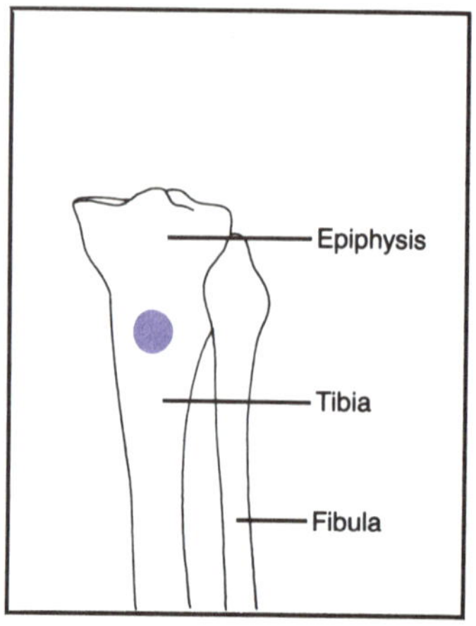

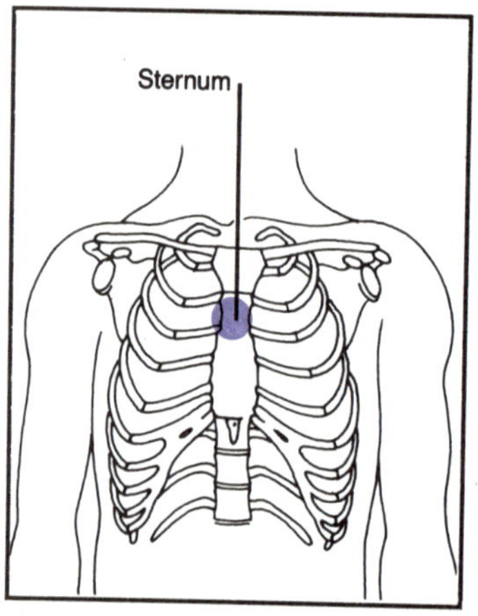

Diagnostic Studies

Other diagnostic tests—*continued*

In an iron stain, decreased hemosiderin levels may indicate a true iron deficiency. Increased levels may accompany other types of anemia or blood disorders. A positive SBB stain can differentiate acute granulocytic leukemia from acute lymphocytic leukemia (SBB-negative) or may indicate granulation in myeloblasts. A positive PAS stain may indicate acute or chronic lymphocytic leukemia, amyloidosis, thalassemia, lymphomas, infectious mononucleosis, iron-deficiency anemia, or sideroblastic anemia.

Nursing considerations. When preparing your patient, describe the procedure and answer any questions. Explain that the test provides a bone marrow specimen for microscopic examination. Inform him that he needn't restrict food or fluids before the test. Tell him who will perform the biopsy, that it usually takes only 5 to 10 minutes, and that test results are usually available in 1 day. Inform him that more than one bone marrow specimen may be necessary and that he'll need to give a blood sample before biopsy for laboratory testing. Check the patient history for a hypersensitivity to the local anesthetic. After checking with the doctor, tell the patient which bone will serve as the biopsy site. Inform him that he'll receive a local anesthetic but that he'll feel pressure on biopsy needle insertion and a brief, pulling pain on marrow removal. As ordered, administer a mild sedative 1 hour before the test. (See *Bone marrow biopsy: Preparing a child,* page 35.)

After the procedure, check the biopsy site for bleeding and inflammation. Observe the patient for signs of hemorrhage and infection—rapid pulse rate, low blood pressure, and fever.

Self-Test

1. Key signs and symptoms of a bleeding disorder include:
1. abnormal bleeding
2. fever
3. enlarged lymph nodes
4. joint pain
a. 1, 2, 3 **b.** 1, 2, 4 **c.** 1, 3, 4 **d.** all of the above

2. An elevated hematocrit level indicates polycythemia or hemodilution.
a. true **b.** false

3. A gallium scan may reveal:
a. Hodgkin's disease **b.** leukemia **c.** thalassemia **d.** Von Willebrand's disease

Answers (page number shows where answer appears in text)
1. **d** (page 9) 2. **b** (page 19) 3. **a** (page 32)

Erythrocyte Disorders: The Anemias and Polycythemias

Dorothy A. Aversa, who wrote this chapter, is an Oncology Nurse in the Research Oncology Department at Mercy Catholic Medical Center, Misericordia Division, Philadelphia. She received her RN diploma from Temple University, Philadelphia.

In this section, which includes Chapters 3 and 4, we'll discuss erythrocyte (red blood cell) disorders (Chapter 3), and leukocyte (white blood cell) disorders (Chapter 4). To build the knowledge base that will enable you to assess your patient thoroughly and intervene appropriately, first review hematopoiesis and erythropoiesis by reading the next few pages.

Hematopoiesis. A continuously self-renewing process, hematopoiesis refers to the formation, production, and maintenance of blood cells in the bone marrow. During fetal life, hematopoiesis starts in the liver and yolk sac, then switches to the bone marrow by the 20th week. By birth, the process occurs in nearly all bones. Fetal hematopoiesis also takes place in the spleen, lymph nodes, and thymus.

Hematopoiesis continues lifelong in the flat bones (the sternum, ribs, vertebrae, and pelvic and shoulder girdles) but slowly declines in long-bone shafts. By age 18, most people show the adult distribution of active bone marrow. With age, fatty tissue replaces inactive marrow, eventually accounting for half of the rib and sternal marrow. Active tissue may replace fatty tissue when blood cell demands increase.

The bone marrow contains self-maintaining pluripotent stem cells (also known as colony-forming units) that can differentiate into erythrocytes, granulocytes, lymphocytes, monocytes, or thrombocytes. Typically, pluripotent stem cells are small, mononuclear, and few in number. The pluripotent cell develops into a committed, or unipotent, stem cell, also called a precursor, progenitor, or early differentiated cell. With the proper stimulus, each unipotent stem cell evolves into a specific cell line. (See *How blood cells evolve.*) Stress can influence this process, stimulating an increase in stem cell production, cell cycle rate, and committed progenitor cells.

Cells made in the bone marrow migrate to the blood. If the body doesn't need them all at once, they move to storage sites, such as the spleen. (For more information, see *Reviewing the spleen's functions.*) Such factors as infection, clotting disorders, cell damage, and ongoing mature cell death influence this continuous process.

Erythropoiesis. This process involves maturation of a nucleated precursor into a hemoglobin-filled, nucleus-free erythrocyte. Regulating the total red blood cell (RBC) mass within precise limits, erythropoiesis ensures that enough cells are available to supply tissues with oxygen but prevents RBC overconcentration, which would impede blood flow through capillaries.

As an RBC precursor matures, it loses its nucleus, leaves the bone marrow through a vein, and circulates in the blood as a *reticulocyte.* After 1 to 4 days, it matures into an erythrocyte—a cell that can withstand the rigors of blood vessel travel—and lives for about 120 days. Approximately 2.5 to 3 million senescent (aged) erythrocytes die each second (normally, a cubic milliliter of blood contains 5 million erythrocytes), necessitating a matching erythrocyte production rate.

Continued on page 40

Reviewing the spleen's functions

The spleen lies below the diaphragm, behind and left of the stomach. Although nonessential for life, the spleen performs these important functions:

- produces erythrocytes in the fetus and, in young children, houses lymphocytes that migrate from the thymus. These lymphocytes' descendants appear in the adult spleen.
- removes and destroys aged or imperfect erythrocytes through phagocytosis, a process known as the culling, or hemoclastic, function
- removes abnormal particles (Howell-Jolly and Heinz bodies) from erythrocytes without destroying the cells, through its pitting function
- stores 20% to 30% of the platelet mass
- breaks down hemoglobin released from destroyed erythrocytes, then returns the iron liberated from hemoglobin catabolism to the bone marrow for reuse
- provides mechanical filtering and antibiotic activity (asplenic patients run an increased risk of sepsis and death).

Erythrocyte Disorders

How blood cells evolve

All blood cells derive from a pluripotent stem cell located in the bone marrow. This cell differentiates into various cells, each of which undergoes further differentiation.

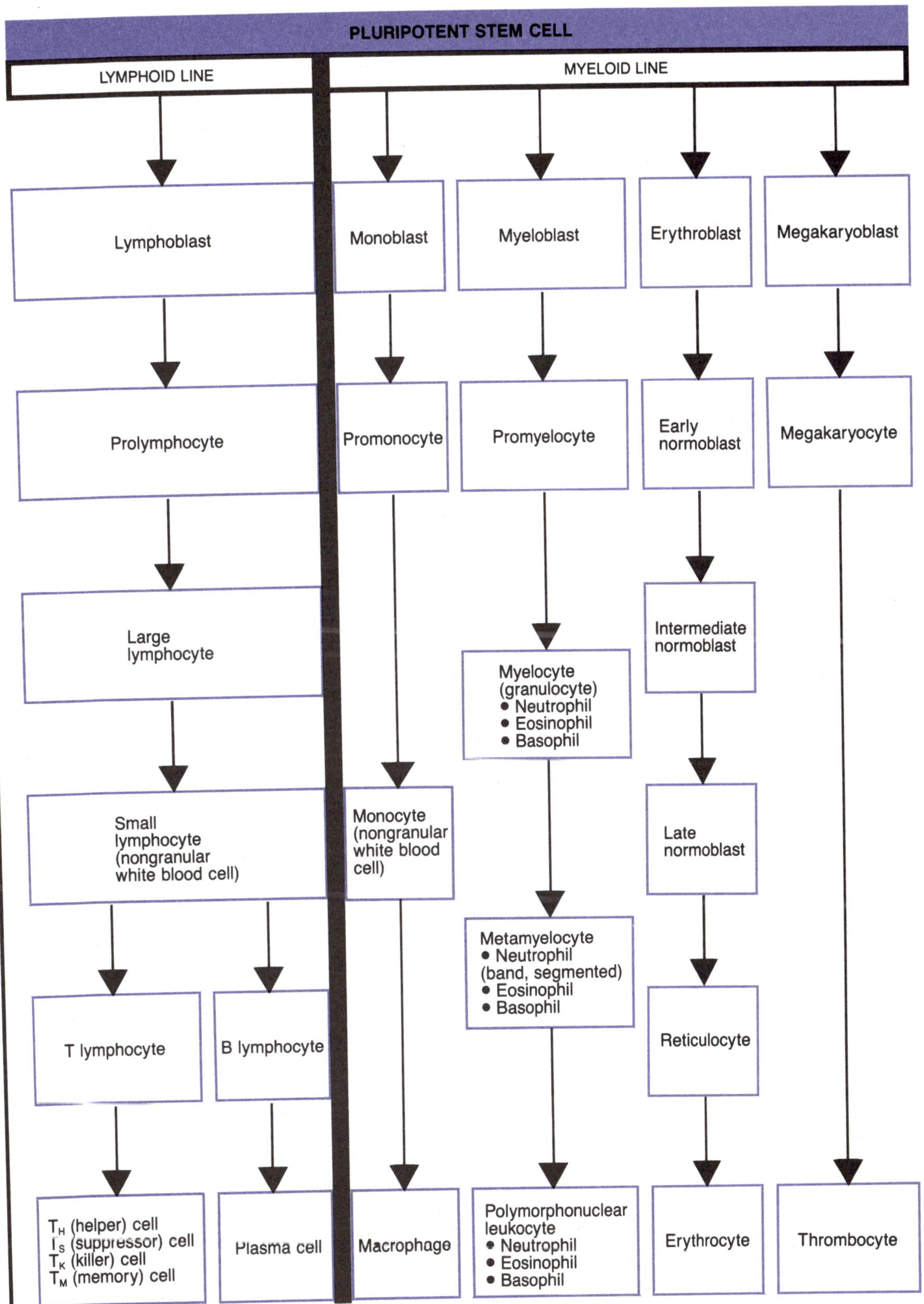

Erythrocyte Disorders

Continued

In an isotonic environment, mature erythrocytes are biconcave disks, measuring about 7 to 8 microns in diameter. Providing a large surface area for gas exchange, this shape also allows flexible movement through narrow capillaries and permits considerable cell expansion without damage.

Tissue oxygen tension mainly controls erythropoiesis. Any condition that causes hypoxia (reduced oxygen transport to tissues)—for example, hemorrhage or living at high altitudes—also increases RBC production by triggering erythropoietin activity (see *How hypoxia stimulates erythropoiesis*). A humoral agent, erythropoietin stimulates RBC production by bone marrow.

The mechanism of erythropoietin formation remains a mystery. Scientists suspect that the kidneys are involved, because patients who've had their kidney removed have only tiny amounts of the substance and usually become anemic from extremely low circulating erythropoietin levels. However, erythropoietin hasn't been isolated from the kidneys. Extrarenal tissues can make small amounts of the substance, and other tissues, such as the liver, appear to make small amounts of the erythropoietin precursor (see *Reviewing the liver's functions*).

When body needs force bone marrow to produce RBCs rapidly, many released cells are immature. The percentage of circulating reticulocytes may then rise as much as 30% to 50% above normal. If the increased demand persists, large numbers of an even less mature cell—the normoblast—may appear. In some serious anemias, normoblasts may account for 5% to 20% of all circulating RBCs. Cells of even less maturity—such as the erythrocyte precursors known as proerythroblasts—may also enter the circulation. Determining the degree of cell immaturity and the number of such immature cells in the bloodstream at any given time helps diagnose anemias.

Erythrocyte abnormalities. Various conditions can cause erythrocyte abnormalities. For example, in a hypertonic environment, erythrocytes shrink as they lose fluid (crenation). In a hypotonic environment, they swell as they gain fluid. With excess fluid gain, their membranes rupture (hemolysis), causing hemoglobin release into surrounding plasma. Certain drugs, snake venoms, and some infections also damage erythrocyte membranes. Other conditions, such as sluggish circulation, cause erythrocytes to adhere like a stack of coins (rouleaux formation) or, as in transfusion reactions, to clump together. These responses can lead to vaso-occlusion and reduce the surface area for gas exchange.

Anemias

The most common erythrocyte disorder, anemia involves a reduction in erythrocyte number, hemoglobin quantity, and packed RBC volume per 100 ml of blood. Consequently, it impairs the blood's oxygen-transporting capacity, causing tissue hypoxia. Some signs and symptoms of anemia stem from compensatory mechanisms triggered by tissue hypoxia (see *Anemia: Compensatory mechnisms*). A clinical sign rather than a specific disease, anemia may arise as a primary

Reviewing the liver's functions

The largest internal organ, the liver lies in the right upper abdominal quadrant. Among its many important hematologic functions, it produces several coagulation substances—fibrinogen, prothrombin, accelerator globulin, and Factors VII, IX, and X. It also contributes to erythropoiesis when bone marrow abnormalities (such as megaloblastic anemia and cancer) occur and during stressful periods.

The liver also converts bilirubin—a hemoglobin end product—to bile. Essential for fat digestion, bile production increases during periods of excessive erythrocyte destruction, as in hemolytic anemia or ineffective erythropoiesis.

The liver also stores iron, first combining it with the protein apoferritin to make ferritin.

Rouleaux formation

When circulation becomes sluggish, red blood cells aggregate like a stack of coins, as shown here.

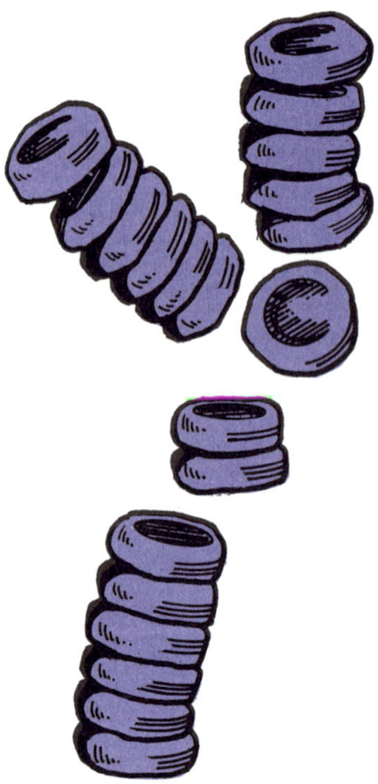

Erythrocyte Disorders

How hypoxia stimulates erythropoiesis

Severe anemia, high altitudes, heart failure, or pulmonary disease causing hypoxemia
↓
Low oxygen concentration in tissues
↓
Hypoxia
↓
Decreased oxygen levels in kidneys and other tissues
↓
Increased renal synthesis of erythropoietin
↓
Increased levels of erythropoietin to bone marrow
↓
Increased bone marrow production of RBCs
↓
Increased oxygen-carrying capacity by hemoglobin
↓
Hypoxia alleviation

Anemia: Compensatory mechanisms

Mechanism
Increased synthesis of 2,3-diphosphoglycerate
Effects
- Increased oxygen release to tissue
- Decreased blood flow to kidneys
- Reduced urine output
- Skin pallor

Mechanism
Increased cardiac output
Effects
- Tachycardia
- Systolic murmur
- Orthostatic hypotension

Mechanism
Increased respiratory rate
Effects
- Exertional dyspnea
- Orthopnea

Mechanism
Increased erythropoietin production
Effects
- Increased RBC production
- Generalized aches and pain
- Sternal tenderness

finding in several disorders—for example, iron, vitamin B_{12}, or folid acid deficiencies; hereditary erythrocyte disorders; bone marrow damage; spleen hyperactivity (hypersplenism); GI tract bleeding; and hemorrhage. Some experts suspect that at least half the world's population suffers from anemia at one time or another. The incidence is especially high in areas with poor nutrition.

Anemias may result from defective erythrocyte production (hypoproliferative anemias) or poor erythrocyte survival (hemolytic anemias). In hypoproliferative anemias, the bone marrow can't produce enough erythrocytes, leading to a reduced reticulocyte count. The problem may stem from drug- or chemical-induced marrow damage or from erythropoietin deficiency. In hemolytic anemias, the problem lies within the erythrocyte itself, the plasma, or the circulation. Whatever the cause, all hemolytic anemias produce an elevated reticulocyte count and a high indirect bilirubin level (sometimes high enough to cause jaundice).

Assessment

Anemia can affect every body system. Here's a list of what to stay alert for when taking your patient's history and performing the physical examination:

- *general*—weight loss, fatigue, depression
- *neurologic system*—headache, syncope, tinnitus, vertigo, cold sensitivity, poor concentration
- *respiratory system*—exertional dyspnea, orthopnea, tachypnea
- *cardiovascular system*—angina, bounding arterial pulses, cardiomegaly, claudication, dependent edema, palpitations, tachycardia, bruits
- *GI system*—anorexia, nausea, diarrhea, constipation, flatulence, splenomegaly
- *genitourinary and reproductive systems*—nocturia, menstrual irregularity, amenorrhea, loss of libido, impotence
- *integumentary system*—pale mucous membranes, nail beds, and palm lines; jaundice; purpura; spider angiomas; pruritus; impaired wound healing
- *musculoskeletal system*—sternal bone tenderness.

Ask the patient whether any family members have suffered anemia. Find out if he has a history of chronic disease, alcohol or drug use, or exposure to industrial or household toxins. Inquire about his diet, which may provide clues to a possible iron, folic acid, or vitamin B_{12} deficiency. Also check for a history of excessive blood loss, such as recent hematemesis, hematuria, or melena.

Diagnostic studies. Expect the doctor to order the following blood studies to help diagnose anemia:

- complete blood count (CBC), which determines the number of blood elements relative to volume and quantifies abnormalities
- blood smear, which identifies RBC color, shape, and size
- hematocrit (HCT) level, or packed cell volume, which measures the RBC percentage per fluid volume of whole blood
- hemoglobin (Hb) level, which measures the amount (in grams) of hemoglobin per 100 ml of blood to determine oxygen-carrying capacity

Continued on page 42

Erythrocyte Disorders

Anemia: Assessing symptom severity

The severity of your patient's anemia symptoms depends on the following factors:

- the speed of anemia's onset—the faster the onset, the worse the symptoms. An otherwise healthy person can tolerate even a 50% decrease in hemoglobin level, RBC count, or hematocrit with few symptoms—if the decrease occurs gradually. However, that same person may experience profound vascular collapse with just a 30% decrease if the decrease occurs rapidly.
- anemia's duration. Someone who's been anemic for a long time probably won't have severe symptoms until his hemoglobin falls to a profoundly subnormal level—2 to 2.5 g/dl. At that point, cardiac failure may occur. With a hemoglobin level between 9 and 11 g/dl, he may have slight tachycardia on exertion. Exertional dyspnea arises when the hemoglobin level drops below 7.5 g/dl; weakness, when it drops below 6 g/dl; and dyspnea at rest, when it falls below 3 g/dl.
- the patient's metabolic requirements. A relatively active person will probably have more symptoms—and more *pronounced* symptoms—than one who's sedentary.
- any concomitant disorders or disabilities. For example, a patient with hypothyroidism may remain asymptomatic even with a hemoglobin level as low as 10 g/dl because he has below-normal oxygen requirements. In contrast, a person with underlying heart disease is more likely than other anemic patients to suffer angina or congestive heart failure, even if he has a higher hemoglobin level.

Anemias—*continued*

- mean corpuscular hemoglobin (MCH), which determines the average amount of hemoglobin per RBC
- mean corpuscular hemoglobin concentration (MCHC), which establishes the average hemoglobin concentration per 100 ml of packed RBCs
- mean corpuscular volume (MCV), which determines RBC size
- reticulocyte count, which assesses RBC production by determining the concentration of this erythrocyte precursor
- Schilling test, which determines absorption of vitamin B_{12} (necessary for erythropoiesis) by measuring radioactive vitamin B_{12} urinary excretion
- sideroblast test, which detects stainable iron (available for hemoglobin synthesis) in normoblastic RBCs
- sugar-water test, which assesses how easily RBCs hemolyze with complement.

Planning

Focus your nursing care on improving the patient's nutritional status, implementing safety measures, ensuring that he gets adequate rest, and teaching him about his disorder.

Nursing diagnoses. Before determining your nursing care plan, develop the nursing diagnosis by identifying the patient's actual or potential problem, then relating it to its cause. Possible nursing diagnoses for the anemic patient include:

- coping, ineffective individual and family (potential for); related to chronic illness
- gas exchange, impaired; related to decreased erythrocyte level and oxygen-carrying capacity of the blood
- nutrition, alteration in (less than body requirements); related to inadequate nutrition
- knowledge deficit; related to diet therapy used in anemia treatment
- activity intolerance; related to fatigue from hypoxia
- mobility, impaired physical; related to weakness and fatigue

Sample nursing care plan: Anemia

Nursing diagnosis	**Expected outcomes**
Coping, ineffective individual and family (potential for); related to chronic illness	The patient will: • express how he feels about having anemia. • explain the underlying cause of his illness. • develop realistic goals. • assist with his care as much as possible.
Nursing interventions	**Discharge planning**
• Teach patient and his family about the disease process and its possible chronic nature. • Schedule time to answer questions. • Review the importance of good nutrition. • Encourage patient to participate in his care as much as possible. • Help patient set realistic goals. • Observe family dynamics to evaluate family's coping mechanisms.	• Consult community health nurse about follow-up care in patient's home, as needed. • Refer patient and his family to a community self-help group for assistance in dealing with chronic disease. • Arrange for follow-up appointments, if needed. • Review patient's care plan with him and his family and answer any questions they may have.

Erythrocyte Disorders

- comfort, alteration in (pain); related to cell sickling or marrow hyperplasia
- self-care deficit; related to impaired physical mobility from extreme weakness
- injury, potential for (trauma); related to fatigue, weakness, or vertigo.

Intervention

Treatment for anemia depends on the specific anemia and its underlying cause. We'll discuss specific treatments later in this chapter, under each anemia type. However, you can refer to the following nursing considerations when caring for any anemic patient.

Help the patient conserve energy. Rest reduces his oxygen requirements, consequently decreasing cardiorespiratory stress. To ensure that he gets adequate rest, keep visits, phone calls, and noise to a minimum. Advise him to lie flat for a few minutes using a pillow if he feels dizzy or light-headed, to increase cerebral perfusion. Encourage the outpatient with mild anemia to take frequent rests throughout the day, to shorten his work day if possible, and to go to bed early.

To find out whether an activity's too strenuous, monitor the patient's pulse as he performs it. If his pulse accelerates rapidly and he develops hypotension, diaphoresis, light-headedness, palpitations, shortness of breath, or weakness, the activity's too strenuous.

If your hospitalized patient has severe anemia, turn him frequently to prevent skin breakdown. (In severe anemia, reduced circulating RBCs greatly limit tissue oxygenation.)

Make sure the patient eats foods high in protein, iron, and vitamins—all essential for erythropoiesis. Teach him and his family how to plan and prepare nourishing meals at home. To help, arrange a consultation with a dietitian and provide booklets on nutrition and meal planning.

If your patient suffers from anorexia brought on by weakness and fatigue, encourage his family to supply his favorite foods (unless he's on a restricted diet). Suggest that someone keep him company as he eats.

An anemic patient may also have a sore mouth, tongue, or esophagus, which makes eating difficult. To help, serve frequent, small meals of soft, cool, bland foods; avoid hot or spicy foods. Clean the patient's teeth with a soft toothbrush before and after meals, and have him rinse his mouth with cool, slightly alkaline mouthwash every 2 hours. Lubricate his lips frequently.

If your patient complains of feeling cold (from poor circulation), use clothing and blankets to warm him. Avoid heating pads and hot water bottles because the anemic patient's oxygen-poor skin burns easily. (The patient may not even feel the burning sensation.)

To decrease the patient's infection risk, use strict aseptic technique. Isolate him from infectious persons, encourage him to wash his

Continued on page 44

Erythrocyte Disorders

Anemias—*continued*

hands often and thoroughly, and advise him to receive necessary immunizations. Before discharge, instruct him to seek medical attention at the first sign of infection.

To prevent complications, watch for signs of bleeding that may exacerbate anemia. Check the patient's stool for occult blood. Assess him for ecchymoses, gingival bleeding, and hematuria. Monitor his vital signs frequently. If he's confined to strict bed rest, help him with range-of-motion exercises, turning, coughing, and deep breathing. Warn him to move about or change positions slowly so he won't get dizzy from cerebral hypoxia.

If your patient needs transfusions to treat severe anemia (hemoglobin level below 5 g/dl), give washed RBCs, as ordered, if pump failure's evident. Monitor for signs and symptoms of circulatory overload or transfusion reaction. Watch for changes in his pulse rate, blood pressure, and respiration. Stay alert for fever, chills, pruritus, or edema. If any of these problems occur, stop the transfusion and notify the doctor. (See *Preparing for a blood transfusion,* page 59; *Blood component therapy,* page 60; and *Recognizing transfusion reactions,* page 61.)

Evaluation

Base your evaluation on the expected outcomes listed on the nursing care plan on page 42. To determine whether your patient has improved, ask yourself such questions as these:

- Has the patient expressed how he feels about having anemia?
- Can he state the cause of his anemia?
- Does he have realistic goals?
- Does he participate in his care?

The answers to these questions will help you evaluate your patient's status and the effectiveness of his care. Remember, these questions stem from the sample care plan on page 42. Your questions may differ.

Hypoproliferative anemias

Among these disorders, we'll discuss aplastic anemia, nutritional deficiency anemias (vitamin B_{12}, folic acid, and iron deficiency anemias), and sideroblastic anemias.

Aplastic anemia

In this disorder, the bone marrow stops making RBCs. Although aplastic anemia can occur alone, it's usually accompanied by granulocytopenia (leukocyte reduction) and thrombocytopenia (thrombocyte reduction)—a condition called *pancytopenia.* Remember—the marrow produces white blood cells (WBCs) and platelets as well as RBCs. Therefore, bone marrow abnormality or damage usually affects the production of all three cell types simultaneously.

Aplastic anemia afflicts about 4 of every million people. It may arise from an unknown cause (about half of all cases) or from such conditions as stem cell damage, bone marrow damage, or immunologic suppression. Specific myelotoxic (marrow-damaging) agents include radiation, benzene, alkylating agents, insecticides, anti-

Erythrocyte Disorders

metabolites, anticonvulsants, chloramphenicol, and sulfonamides. These agents may exert a metabolic effect on cellular differentiation or trigger an autoimmune response against immature hematopoietic precursor cells.

Aplastic anemia may have a rapid or a gradual onset. Myelotoxin-induced bone marrow failure may produce an explosive onset, whereas idiopathic anemia typically arises gradually.

Assessment. The patient with aplastic anemia usually complains of progressive fatigue, lassitude, and dyspnea. The blood smear shows a normocytic anemia. The WBC differential reveals granulocytopenia, indicating an increased susceptibility to infection. The platelet count reveals thrombocytopenia, suggesting an increased bleeding disorder risk.

Intervention. The doctor will base treatment on the disorder's severity. As ordered, discontinue any potentially toxic agent. (A patient who's receiving treatment with a myelotoxin should have frequent hemograms.)

The doctor will probably order blood transfusions for a patient whose anemia causes disability or life-threatening bleeding. Continue the transfusion only until bone marrow resumes RBC production (or as ordered). Unnecessary transfusion increases the risk of immune reactions to platelets, shortens platelet life span, and may speed the rejection rate of transplanted marrow cells. Repeated transfusions can also cause hemosiderosis and an enlarged spleen. (See *Preparing for a blood transfusion,* page 59; *Blood component therapy,* page 60; and *Recognizing transfusion reactions,* page 61.) For a severely anemic patient who needs frequent transfusions, the doctor may order chelating agents to remove excess iron. Splenectomy may prove necessary for the patient with an enlarged spleen that leads to destruction of normal RBCs or suppression of RBC development in bone marrow.

Corticosteroids and androgens may help stimulate bone marrow function; transfused platelet concentrates may correct life-threatening thrombocytopenia. To reduce the chance that antiplatelet antibodies impair platelet effectiveness, pay careful attention to human leukocyte antigen typing of donor platelets.

Scientists are currently studying a treatment involving marrow mixed with a soybean protein that isolates mature lymphocytes, facilitating their removal. The patient would then receive the remaining immature lymphocytes, which would acquire tolerance to his tissues and function normally.

Bone marrow transplantation may be practical for a patient who has a matched donor. Successful transplantation can allow the patient to lead a normal life; however, the procedure can cause fatal complications. (See Chapter 4 for details on bone marrow transplantation.)

Nursing interventions. Consider the most important part of your care correcting or preventing infection and bleeding—major pancytopenia complications.

Continued on page 46

Erythrocyte Disorders

Hypoproliferative anemias—*continued*

If your patient already has an infection, assess him every 4 hours for signs and symptoms of worsening infection. These include:
- a temperature increase
- mouth lesions, color changes, tongue soreness and swelling
- rectal tenderness, redness, induration, and hemorrhoids
- constipation or diarrhea
- skin redness, swelling, induration, lesions, and pain
- painful breathing, cough, adventitious breath sounds, and shortness of breath
- dysuria and foul-smelling urine
- I.V. site redness, swelling, tenderness, and pain.

Be sure to control environmental factors that can contribute to infection. Practice strict hand washing. Keep flowers, fresh fruits, and vegetables out of the patient's room; remove vases or other sources of standing water. Screen visitors and staff for fever, nausea, vomiting, colds, and varicella. Provide masks for those with upper respiratory infections. If your patient's in a private room, keep the door closed. Use strict aseptic technique, including masks for you and the patient, when suctioning, changing dressings, and changing pressure monitor lines and central I.V. tubing. Also, make sure the housekeeping staff damp-dusts, washes the floor, and cleans countertops with disinfectant daily.

To help safeguard your patient's immune responses, turn and position him every hour. Bathe him daily with mild soap and warm water to keep his skin clean. Apply lotion every 3 to 4 hours to keep his skin well lubricated. Once each shift, make sure a nurse checks the patient's skin turgor to assess his hydration status. Keep a humidifier in the patient's room.

Change soiled or wet linens. Implement chest physiotherapy as needed. If your patient's immobile, help him perform range-of-motion exercises every 4 hours. Also have him cough and breathe deeply and perform incentive spirometry every 4 hours.

To help prevent bleeding and infection, avoid invasive procedures, such as enemas, injections, and rectal temperature checks. Instruct the patient to avoid trauma—for instance, by using an electric razor and avoiding straining during defecation. Tell him to report any signs or symptoms of infection.

(For guidelines on caring for the patient with a bleeding disorder, read Chapters 5 and 6.)

Vitamin B_{12} deficiency anemia

Also known as pernicious anemia, vitamin B_{12} deficiency anemia involves decreased gastric production of hydrochloric acid and intrinsic factor (IF). Normally secreted by gastric mucosal parietal cells, IF plays a key role in vitamin B_{12} absorption.

The familial incidence of vitamin B_{12} deficiency anemia suggests a genetic predisposition. Most experts believe this anemia's caused by an inherited autoimmune response that leads to gastric mucosal atrophy, decreasing hydrochloric acid and IF production. Patients with immunologically related disorders, such as thyroiditis, myx-

Erythrocyte Disorders

edema, and Graves' disease, have a significantly higher incidence of this anemia.

Vitamin B_{12} deficiency anemia can cause serious hematologic abnormalities, including inhibited growth of all cells—particularly RBCs; this leads to insufficient and deformed RBCs with fragile membranes and poor oxygen-carrying capacity. The cardiovascular system attempts to compensate by increasing cardiac output, which can trigger various problems.

Vitamin B_{12} deficiency anemia also causes demyelination (impaired myelin formation), resulting in neurologic damage. Demyelination typically spreads from peripheral nerves to the spinal cord. Although some neurologic signs and symptoms are temporary, irreversible neurologic changes can occur before the patient seeks treatment. Left untreated, this anemia may lead to permanent neurologic disability and death.

Vitamin B_{12} deficiency anemia primarily affects persons of northern European ancestry. It's rare among children, blacks, and Asians. Typically, the disease occurs between ages 50 and 60; its incidence rises with increasing age.

Assessment. Although it usually has an insidious onset, vitamin B_{12} deficiency anemia eventually causes an unmistakable symptom triad: weakness, sore tongue, and numbness and tingling in the arms and legs. The lips, tongue, and gums appear bloodless. Hemolysis-induced hyperbilirubinemia may cause faintly jaundiced sclera and pale to bright yellow skin. The patient may suffer frequent infections, especially of the genitourinary tract.

When assessing a patient for this anemia, check for indications of a below-normal hemoglobin level—for example, weakness, fatigue, light-headedness, palpitations, wide pulse pressure, dyspnea, orthopnea, tachycardia, premature beats, and congestive heart failure.

GI problems, caused by gastric mucosal atrophy and reduced hydrochloric acid production, may include digestive disturbances, nausea, vomiting, anorexia, weight loss, flatulence, diarrhea, and constipation. Gingival bleeding and tongue inflammation may intensify anorexia.

Also check for neurologic problems resulting from demyelination—for example, neuritis, extremity weakness, peripheral numbness and paresthesias, disturbed position sense, incoordination, ataxia, impaired fine finger movement, positive Babinski's and Romberg's signs, light-headedness, disturbed vision (diplopia, blurriness), tinnitus, altered taste, optic muscle atrophy, bowel and bladder incontinence, impotence, irritability, poor memory, headache, and depression.

Findings from blood studies, bone marrow aspiration, and gastric analysis help establish the diagnosis. The Schilling test proves definitive. (See *Schilling test* for more details.) Laboratory screening tests must rule out other anemias (such as folic acid deficiency anemia) that cause similar symptoms because treatment differs.

Continued on page 48

Schilling test

An indirect analysis of intrinsic factor (IF) deficiency, the Schilling test evaluates vitamin B_{12} absorption from the GI tract by measuring radioactive vitamin B_{12} excreted in the urine. A 24-hour urine test, it helps differentiate vitamin B_{12} deficiency anemia and malabsorption syndrome.

The patient first receives a small (0.5- to 2-mcg) oral dose of radioactive vitamin B_{12} after fasting for 12 hours. Two hours later, he receives a 1-mcg dose of *nonradioactive* vitamin B_{12} I.M., as a parenteral flush. Urine is collected for 24 hours, then evaluated for radioactive vitamin B_{12}.

A normal healthy person excretes about 8% or more of the radioactive vitamin in his urine. Below-normal (0% to 3%) excretion may mean IF deficiency or defective vitamin B_{12} absorption in the ileum.

To rule out intestinal malabsorption, the doctor will repeat the Schilling test, this time adding IF. If urinary excretion then rises to a normal level, the patient probably has an IF deficiency, suggesting vitamin B_{12} deficiency anemia. Urinary excretion that fails to rise suggests a malabsorption syndrome. (However, patients with diabetes, hypothyroidism, or enteritis normally have depressed urinary excretion, as do many elderly patients.)

Nursing considerations. Explain the test's purpose and procedure to the patient. Remind him to fast and collect his urine for the prescribed period. (Be sure to let him know he can drink water throughout this period.)

After the patient receives the first I.M. vitamin B_{12} dose, he can have foods and fluids; encourage him to drink as much as he can during the 24-hour test period. Avoid administering laxatives during that time.

Erythrocyte Disorders

Hypoproliferative anemias—*continued*

Diagnostic tests must also rule out vitamin B_{12} deficiency resulting from malabsorption caused by GI disorders, gastric surgery, radiation, or drug therapy.

Blood test results that suggest vitamin B_{12} deficiency anemia include:

- decreased hemoglobin (4 to 5 g/dl) and RBC levels
- increased MCV (above 120) and increased MCHC resulting from the increased hemoglobin content of larger than normal RBCs
- possibly low WBC and platelet counts
- large, malformed platelets
- serum vitamin B_{12} assay levels below 0.1 mcg/ml
- elevated lactic dehydrogenase level.

Bone marrow aspiration reveals erythroid hyperplasia (crowded red bone marrow) with increased numbers of megaloblasts but few normally developing RBCs. Gastric analysis shows absence of free hydrochloric acid after histamine or pentagastrin injection.

Intervention. Early parenteral vitamin B_{12} replacement can reverse vitamin B_{12} deficiency anemia and minimize complications and may prevent permanent neurologic damage. Expect the doctor to order an initial high dose of parenteral vitamin B_{12} to permit rapid RBC regeneration. Within 2 weeks, the hemoglobin level should rise to normal and the patient's condition should improve visibly. Because rapid cell regeneration increases iron requirements, the patient will need concomitant iron replacement to prevent iron deficiency anemia.

After the patient's condition improves, the doctor will probably lower the vitamin B_{12} dose to a maintenance level, given monthly. Because these injections must continue for life, teach the patient self-administration.

An extremely fatigued patient may require bed rest until his hemoglobin level rises. With a dangerously low hemoglobin level, the patient may need blood transfusions, digitalis, a diuretic, and a low-sodium diet to prevent or control congestive heart failure. Vitamin B_{12} replacement helps manage the condition that led to this failure. As ordered, administer antibiotics to help combat accompanying infections.

Nursing interventions. Teach your patient and his family about vitamin B_{12} deficiency anemia. Emphasize that vitamin B_{12} replacement doesn't cure the disease and that these injections must continue for life, even after symptoms subside.

If your patient's severely anemic, schedule activities, rest periods, and necessary diagnostic tests to conserve his energy. Monitor his pulse rate often; tachycardia means that his activities are too strenuous. Also warn the patient to guard against infection and to promptly report infection symptoms.

If neurologic damage causes behavioral problems, assess the patient's mental and neurologic status often. If necessary, give tranquilizers, as ordered, and apply a jacket restraint at night.

Erythrocyte Disorders

Provide a well-balanced diet, including foods high in vitamin B_{12} (meat, liver, fish, eggs, and milk). Offer the patient between-meal snacks and encourage his family to bring his favorite foods from home. If he has a sore mouth and tongue, ask the dietitian to provide only cool, bland foods. Supply diluted mouthwash or, with severe conditions, swab the patient's mouth with tap water or warm saline solution. Mouth lesions may also make talking difficult. If so, provide a pad and pencil for communication.

Warn the patient with a sensory deficit not to use a heating pad because it may cause burns. With an incontinent patient, establish a regular bowel and bladder routine. Arrange for a visiting nurse to follow up on this schedule and make adjustments, if necessary, after discharge.

To *prevent* vitamin B_{12} deficiency anemia, emphasize the importance of vitamin B_{12} supplements for patients who've had extensive gastric resections or who follow strict vegetarian diets.

Folic acid deficiency anemia
A common and slowly progressive anemia, folic acid deficiency anemia occurs most often in infants, adolescents, pregnant and lactating women, alcoholics, elderly persons, and those with cancer or intestinal disease. The disorder may result from alcohol abuse (because alcohol suppresses folic acid's metabolic effects), poor diet (common in alcoholics, elderly persons living alone, and infants, especially those with infection or diarrhea), impaired absorption (as with celiac disease, tropical sprue, regional jejunitis, or bowel resection), bacteria competing for available folic acid, and prolonged drug therapy with anticonvulsants and estrogens. Excessive cooking, which destroys much of the folic acid in foods, can also be a factor. The rapid growth of infants increases the folic acid requirement, as do pregnancy, lactation, and some neoplastic and skin diseases. (Infants may suffer from this anemia because they have a limited folic acid storage capacity.) In children and adolescents, an increased folic acid requirement may stem from drinking folate-poor cow's milk.

Assessment. When assessing your patient, keep in mind that folic acid deficiency anemia gradually produces clinical features characteristic of severe vitamin B_{12} deficiency anemia, without the neurologic manifestations. Check for such typical signs and symptoms as progressive fatigue, shortness of breath, palpitations, weakness, glossitis, nausea, anorexia, headache, fainting, irritability, forgetfulness, pallor, and slight jaundice.

Expect the doctor to order the Schilling test and a therapeutic trial of vitamin B_{12} injections to distinguish between folic acid and vitamin B_{12} deficiency anemia. Significant blood findings include macrocytosis, decreased reticulocyte count, abnormal platelets, and a serum folate level below 4 mg/ml.

Intervention. Treatment consists mainly of folic acid supplements and elimination of contributing causes. As ordered, give folic acid supplements orally or parenterally. Parenteral administration usually proves necessary for severely ill patients who can't take oral medication. Many patients respond favorably to a well-balanced diet.

Continued on page 50

Erythrocyte Disorders

Foods high in folic acid

Folic acid (pteroylglutamic acid, folacin) is found in most body tissues, where it acts as a coenzyme in metabolic processes involving one carbon transfer. It's essential for RBC formation and maturation and for deoxyribonucleic acid synthesis. Although its body stores are comparatively small (about 70 mg), this vitamin's plentiful in most well-balanced diets.

However, because it's water-soluble and heat-labile, it's easily destroyed by cooking. Also, approximately 20% of folic acid intake is excreted unabsorbed. Insufficient daily folic acid intake (<50 mcg/day) usually induces folic acid deficiency within 4 months. Here's a list of foods high in folic acid content.

Food	Folic acid content (mcg/100 g)
Asparagus spears	109
Beef liver	294
Broccoli spears	54
Collards (cooked)	102
Mushrooms	24
Oatmeal	33
Peanut butter	57
Red beans	180
Wheat germ	305

Hypoproliferative anemias—*continued*

Nursing intervention. Teach the patient to meet his daily folic acid requirements by including a food from each food group in every meal. Explain to the severely deficient patient that diet only reinforces folic acid supplementation and isn't therapeutic by itself. Encourage your patient to comply with prescribed therapy and advise him to continue taking supplements even when he begins to feel better.

If the patient has glossitis, emphasize the importance of good oral hygiene. Suggest regular use of mild or diluted mouthwash and a soft toothbrush.

Monitor fluid and electrolyte status, particularly in the patient with severe diarrhea who's receiving parenteral fluid replacement therapy.

Remember that anemia causes severe fatigue. Schedule regular rest periods until the patient can resume normal activity.

To *prevent* folic acid deficiency anemia, emphasize the importance of a well-balanced diet high in folic acid (see *Foods high in folic acid*). Identify alcoholics with poor dietary habits, and try to arrange for appropriate counseling. Advise mothers who aren't breast-feeding to feed their babies commercially prepared formulas.

Iron-deficiency anemia
This anemia occurs when the body's iron stores prove inadequate for optimal erythropoiesis, resulting in small (microcytic) RBCs with less color on staining (see *Iron absorption and storage*). The plasma iron level and the plasma transferrin level decrease (transferrin binds with and transports iron). Ultimately, this leads to a depleted RBC mass and, in turn, to decreased hemoglobin concentration levels (hypochromia) and reduced blood oxygen-carrying capacity.

A common disease worldwide, iron-deficiency anemia affects 10% to 30% of American adults, occurring most commonly in premenopausal women, infants (particularly premature or low-birth-weight infants), children, and adolescents (especially girls).

Iron-deficiency anemia can result from the following:
- an iron-poor diet, containing less than 2 mg/day, as in prolonged unsupplemented breast- or bottle-feeding of infants and during stressful periods, such as rapid childhood and adolescent growth
- iron malabsorption, as in chronic diarrhea, partial or total gastrectomy, and malabsorption syndromes such as celiac disease
- blood loss secondary to drug-induced GI bleeding (from anticoagulants, aspirin, or steroids) or from heavy menses, trauma-induced hemorrhage, GI ulcers, cancer, or varices
- pregnancy, in which the mother's iron supply is diverted to the fetus for erythropoiesis
- intravascular hemolysis-induced hemoglobinuria or paroxysmal nocturnal hemoglobinuria
- mechanical erythrocyte trauma caused by a prosthetic heart valve.

Assessment. Because it progresses gradually, iron-deficiency anemia rarely causes early signs and symptoms. Consequently, patients

Erythrocyte Disorders

Iron absorption and storage

Iron, essential to erythropoiesis, is abundant throughout the body. Two thirds of total body iron exists in hemoglobin; the other third, mostly in the mononuclear phagocytic system (liver, spleen, bone marrow), with small amounts in muscle, blood serum, and body cells.

Adequate dietary ingestion of iron and recirculation of iron released from disintegrating RBCs maintain iron supplies. The duodenum and upper part of the small intestine absorb dietary iron. Such absorption depends on gastric acid content, the amount of reducing substances (ascorbic acid, for example) in the alimentary canal, and dietary iron intake. With deficient iron intake, the body gradually depletes its iron stores, causing decreased hemoglobin levels and, eventually, signs and symptoms of iron-deficiency anemia.

typically seek medical treatment only when the condition becomes severe. A classic sign is *pica*—the desire to eat nonfood items. For example, the patient may crave ice (pacophagia) or dirt (geophagia).

In advanced iron-deficiency anemia, the patient has dyspnea on exertion, fatigue, listlessness, pallor, poor concentration, irritability, headache, and susceptibility to infection. Decreased oxygen perfusion causes the heart to compensate with increased cardiac output and tachycardia.

In the patient with chronic iron-deficiency anemia, nails become spoon-shaped and brittle, mouth corners crack, the tongue turns smooth, and dysphagia occurs. Associated neuromuscular effects include vasomotor disturbances, arm and leg numbness and tingling, and neuralgic pain.

The doctor will order blood studies (such as serum iron, total iron-binding capacity, and ferritin levels) and bone marrow studies to help confirm iron-deficiency anemia. However, complicating factors, such as infection, pneumonia, blood transfusion, and iron supplements, can make test findings misleading. The doctor must also rule out other anemia forms, such as those resulting from thalassemia minor, cancer, and chronic inflammatory, hepatic, or renal disease.

Characteristic blood findings include the following:
- subnormal hemoglobin level (males, below 12 g/dl; females, below 10 g/dl)
- subnormal hematocrit level (males, below 47 ml/dl; females, below 42 ml/dl)
- subnormal serum iron level, with high binding capacity
- subnormal serum ferritin level
- decreased RBC count, with microcytic and hypochromic cells (in early anemia, the RBC count may appear normal, except in infants and children)
- decreased MCH (in severe anemia).

Bone marrow studies reveal normoblastic hyperplasia. With staining, they show depleted or absent iron stores.

Intervention. Once iron deficiency has been identified as anemia's underlying cause, the doctor will probably order replacement therapy. Most patients can take oral preparations of iron or iron and ascorbic acid, which enhances iron absorption. However, your patient may need parenteral iron administration if he won't take the oral preparation, if he needs more iron than he can take orally, or if he has a malabsorption syndrome that prevents adequate iron absorption from the GI tract. The doctor may also order parenteral iron administration to achieve a maximum hemoglobin regeneration rate.

Because total-dose I.V. infusion of supplemental iron is painless and requires fewer injections, it's usually preferable to I.M. administration. Pregnant patients and geriatric patients with severe anemia, for example, should receive a total-dose infusion of iron dextran in normal saline solution over 8 hours. To minimize the risk of an allergic reaction, first give the patient an I.V. test dose of 0.5 ml.

Continued on page 52

Erythrocyte Disorders

Injecting iron solutions

For deep I.M. injections of iron solutions (such as iron dextran), use the Z-track technique to avoid subcutaneous irritation and discoloration from leaking medication. Choose a 19G or 20G, 5- to 7.5-cm (2″ to 3″) needle. After drawing up the solution, change to a fresh needle to avoid tracking the solution through to subcutaneous tissue. Allow 0.5 ml of air into the syringe.

Displace the skin, fat, and muscle at the injection site (in the buttocks' upper outer quadrant only) firmly to one side. Cleanse the area, and insert the needle. Aspirate to check for entry into a blood vessel. Inject the solution slowly, followed by the 0.5 ml of air in the syringe. Wait 10 seconds, pull the needle straight out, and release the tissues.

Apply direct pressure to the site, but don't massage it. Caution the patient against vigorous exercise for 15 to 30 minutes.

Injection sites

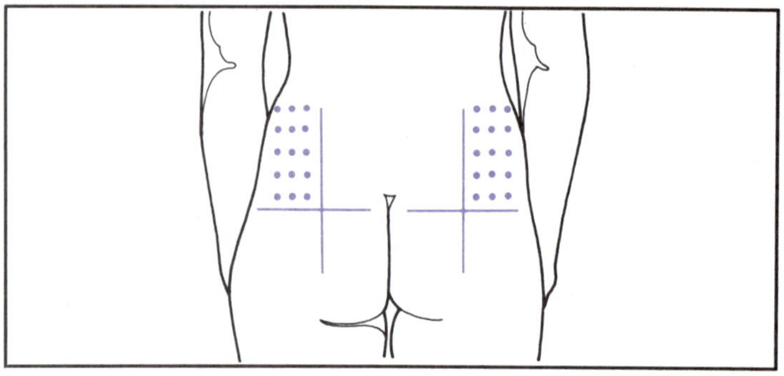

1. Displace tissues.

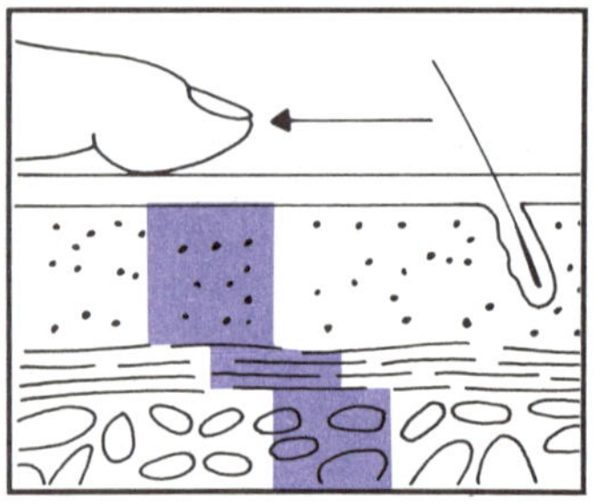

2. Inject solution.

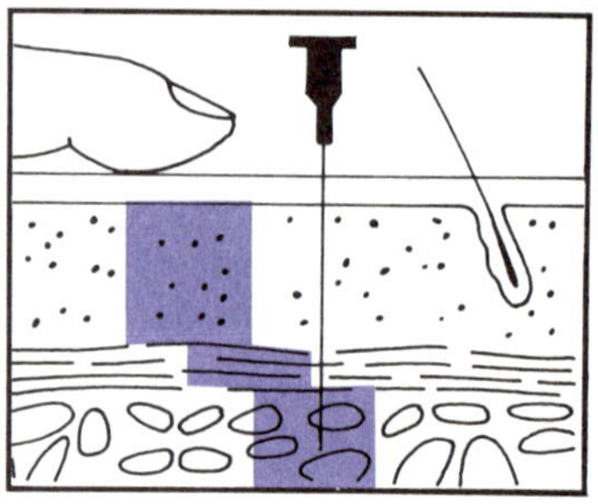

3. Wait 10 seconds.

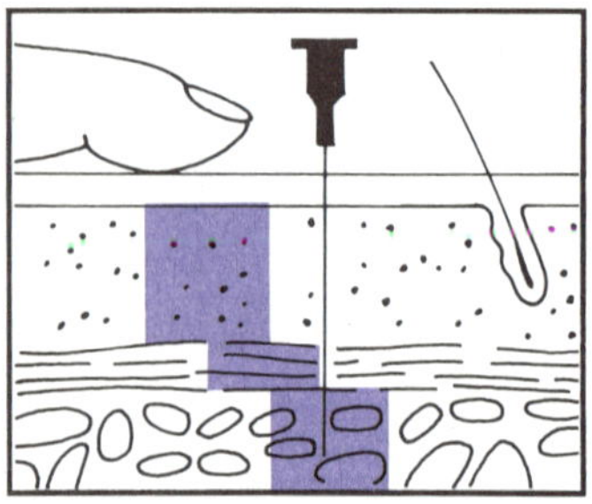

4. Release tissues.

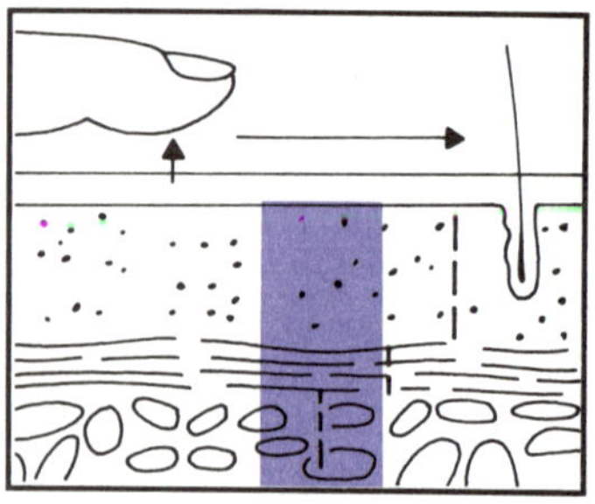

Hypoproliferative anemias—*continued*

Nursing intervention. Monitor the patient's compliance with the prescribed iron supplement therapy. Advise him not to stop therapy even if he feels better, because iron replenishment takes time. Explain that milk and antacids interfere with iron absorption, whereas vitamin C can increase iron absorption. Instruct him to drink liquid

Erythrocyte Disorders

supplemental iron through a straw so that it won't stain his teeth. Tell him to report any adverse effects of iron therapy, such as nausea, vomiting, diarrhea, or constipation, which may necessitate a dosage adjustment.

If the patient's receiving I.V. iron supplements, monitor the infusion rate carefully and watch for an allergic response. Stop the infusion and begin supportive treatment if he shows signs or symptoms of an adverse reaction. Also watch for dizziness and headache and for thrombophlebitis around the I.V. site.

When administering iron I.M., use the Z-track injection method to prevent skin discoloration, scarring, and irritating iron deposits. (See *Injecting iron solutions.*)

Because iron deficiency can recur, advise your patient to have regular checkups.

To *prevent* iron-deficiency anemia, teach patients about the basics of a nutritionally balanced diet—red meats, green vegetables, eggs, whole wheat products, iron-fortified bread, and milk. Assess the patient's drug history. Some drugs, such as pancreatic enzymes and vitamin E, may interfere with iron metabolism and absorption. Such drugs as aspirin and steroids may cause GI bleeding. Teach a patient who must take such gastric irritants to take them with meals or milk.

Emphasize the need for high-risk individuals—premature infants, children under age 2, adolescents, and pregnant women—to receive prophylactic oral iron, as ordered. (Children under age 2 should also receive supplemental high-iron cereals and formulas.)

Assess a family's diet for iron content and note the influence of childhood eating patterns, cultural food preferences, and family income. Encourage families with deficient iron intake to eat meat, fish, poultry, whole or enriched grain products, and foods high in ascorbic acid.

Ringed sideroblast

Electron microscopy, illustrated here, shows large iron deposits in the mitochondria, forming the characteristic ringed sideroblast in sideroblastic anemias.

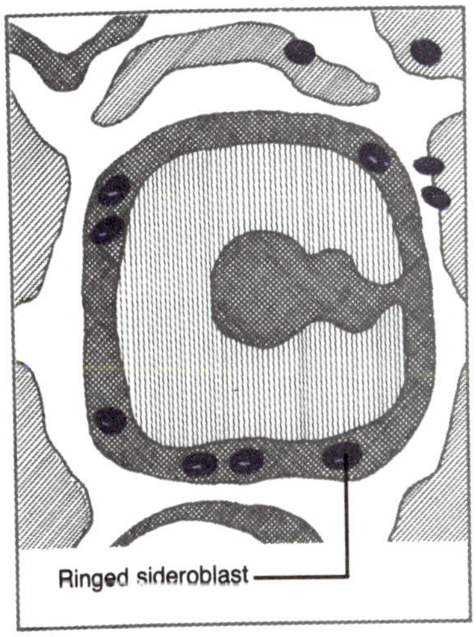

Sideroblastic anemias

These chronic disorders are characterized by hyperplastic erythroid bone marrow containing many iron-laden, developing normoblasts (erythrocyte precursors). Known as sideroblasts, such normoblasts fail to use iron to synthesize hemoglobin. As a result, iron accumulates in the mitochondria (see *Ringed sideroblast*).

Sideroblastic anemias may be hereditary or acquired; the acquired form can be primary or secondary. Hereditary sideroblastic anemia appears to follow an X-linked inheritance pattern and occurs mostly in young males. Females are carriers and rarely show signs of the disorder.

The primary acquired form most commonly affects elderly persons but occasionally develops in the young. While its cause remains unknown, it typically appears in conjunction with thrombocytopenia or leukopenia. The secondary acquired form may stem from exposure to or ingestion of toxins, such as alcohol and lead, or use of drugs, such as isoniazid and chloramphenicol. This form can also

Continued on page 54

Erythrocyte Disorders

Hypoproliferative anemias—*continued*

occur as a complication of other diseases, such as rheumatoid arthritis, lupus erythematosus, plasma cell myeloma, tuberculosis, and severe infection.

Assessment. The patient with sideroblastic anemia usually has nonspecific clinical signs and symptoms, which may remain unidentified for several years. Assess your patient for anorexia, fatigue, weakness, dizziness, skin and mucous membrane pallor, and enlarged lymph nodes. Heart and liver failure, which may develop from excessive iron accumulation in these organs, can cause dyspnea, exertional angina, slight jaundice, and hepatosplenomegaly. A patient with hereditary sideroblastic anemia usually has increased GI iron absorption, causing signs of hemosiderosis (abnormal iron deposition in body tissues). Findings typical of the secondary form depend on the underlying condition.

Expect the doctor to order microscopic examination of bone marrow aspirate, stained with Prussian blue or alizarin dye, which typically reveals ringed sideroblasts. Microscopic blood examination shows hypochromic or normochromic and slightly enlarged erythrocytes. Erythrocyte precursors may appear megaloblastic, with anisocytosis (abnormal size variation) and poikilocytosis (abnormal shape variation). Unlike iron-deficiency anemia, sideroblastic anemia lowers the hemoglobin level and raises serum iron and transferrin levels. In turn, faulty hemoglobin production increases urobilinogen and bilirubin levels. Platelet and leukocyte levels remain normal, but thrombocytopenia or leukopenia may occur.

Intervention. Treatment depends on the anemia's underlying cause. The hereditary form usually responds to several weeks of pyridoxine (vitamin B_6) treatment. The secondary acquired form usually subsides after elimination of the causative drug or toxin or with correction of the underlying condition. Folic acid supplements may also prove helpful when erythrocyte precursors show concomitant megaloblastic nuclear changes.

The primary acquired form resists treatment. Patients usually die within 10 years of the appearance of complications (especially respiratory and cardiac problems) or concomitant disease (usually acute leukemia). Elderly patients are less likely to improve and stand a greater chance of developing serious complications. Deferoxamine mesylate may prove useful for treating chronic iron overload. For some patients with the primary acquired form, the doctor may order carefully cross-matched transfusions to provide needed hemoglobin or high androgen doses as a palliative measure. He may also order phlebotomy to prevent hemochromatosis. Phlebotomy speeds the erythropoiesis rate and uses up excess iron, reducing the serum and total-body iron burden.

Nursing intervention. Administer prescribed medications and teach the patient the importance of continuing with drug therapy even after he begins to feel better. Provide frequent rest periods if he becomes easily fatigued.

Erythrocyte Disorders

If the patient's scheduled for phlebotomy, explain the procedure. If several such procedures prove necessary, provide a high-protein diet to help replace lost protein. Encourage the patient to follow a similar diet at home.

Find out about possible lead exposure in the home (especially for young children) or on the job. If your patient abuses alcohol, refer him for therapy.

Hemolytic anemias

A shortened erythrocyte life span characterizes these anemias. The bone marrow tries to compensate by accelerating erythrocyte production—in some cases, to more than three times the normal rate. Consequently, hemolytic anemias cause an elevated reticulocyte count, an increased indirect bilirubin fraction, and a subnormal haptoglobin (hemoglobin-binding protein) level.

Hemolytic anemias can be acquired or inherited. For information on the acquired forms, see *Acquired hemolytic anemias: Identifying underlying causes.* For information on the inherited forms—hereditary spherocytosis, sickle-cell anemia, and the thalassemias—read on.

Hereditary spherocytosis

A common form of chronic hemolytic anemia, hereditary spherocytosis occurs in persons of all ages and races. It's inherited as an autosomal dominant trait. Large numbers of spherocytes—sphere-shaped erythrocytes—and an enlarged spleen characterize the disorder. Spherocytes have defective membranes, making them extremely permeable to sodium. In an attempt to stop sodium ion flow into its cytoplasm, the cell steps up its metabolic output, using too much glucose. Eventually, the cell wears out and sodium ions flow in unchecked. The interior then becomes hypertonic and, as water enters, the cell swells.

Continued on page 56

Acquired hemolytic anemias: Identifying underlying causes

Disorder	Cause	Assessment findings
Heart valve hemolysis	RBC damage from regurgitant flow through an incompetent valve prosthesis	Fragmented RBCs
Immune hemolytic anemia	Antibodies, sometimes secondary to administration of such drugs as methyldopa and penicillin	Jaundice, spherocytes
Microangiopathic hemolytic anemia	RBC damage from flow through abnormal, small blood vessels, as in malignant hypertension	Fragmented RBCs
Paroxysmal nocturnal hemoglobinuria	Unknown; occasionally follows aplastic anemia	Hemoglobinuria, especially in the morning; possible pancytopenia; multiple venous thrombosis
Spur-cell anemia	Severe liver disease (usually portal hypertension); increased lipids in RBC membrane	Spur-shaped RBCs

Sickle-cell anemia inheritance patterns

As this chart shows, in only two situations can you predict the outcome with certainty.

The first and most serious risk occurs when both parents have sickle-cell anemia; childbearing—if possible at all—may prove dangerous for the mother, and all offspring will have sickle-cell anemia.

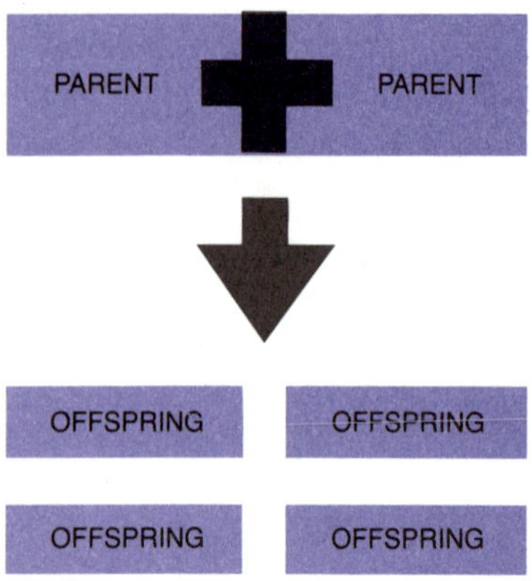

When one parent has sickle-cell anemia and one is normal, all offspring will be sickle-cell anemia carriers.

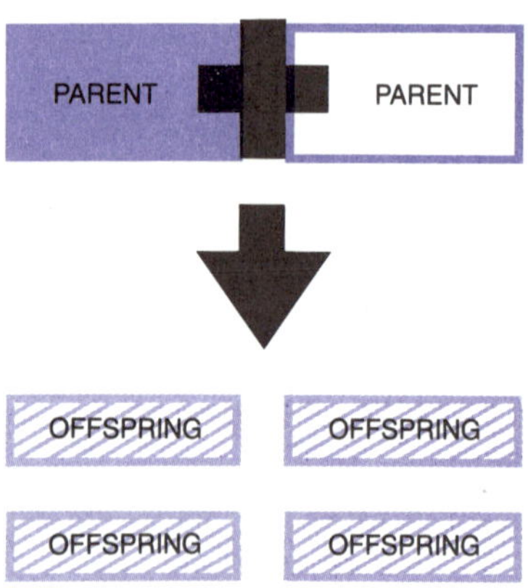

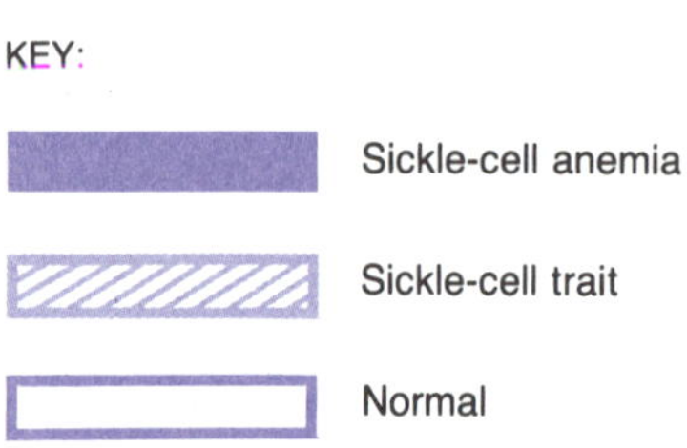

Hemolytic anemias—*continued*

Thick and relatively inflexible, spherocytes easily become trapped inside the spleen. As a result, the spleen enlarges as its phagocytes remove the abnormal cells. Massive hemolysis in the spleen then causes anemia and jaundice.

Assessment. Hereditary spherocytosis causes signs and symptoms typical of other hemolytic anemias—malaise; jaundice; and splenomegaly, which results in left upper quadrant pain and a feeling of fullness.

Typical laboratory findings include spherocytes in the blood smear, reticulocytosis, and subnormal hemoglobin and RBC levels. The spherocyte's smaller surface area and larger content cause increased osmotic fragility (spherocytes rupture quickly when placed in hypotonic saline solution).

Intervention. Although hereditary spherocytosis can't be cured, it can be treated by splenectomy, which completely reverses symptoms in 90% of patients. Although spherocytes continue to circulate after spleen removal, they have a normal or near-normal life span. Blood transfusions may help the patient who's in hemolytic crisis.

Sickle-cell anemia

This chronic hereditary disorder exists in both an anemia form and a trait form (see *Sickle-cell anemia inheritance patterns*). It results from a defective hemoglobin molecule (hemoglobin S). Upon erythrocyte deoxygenation (which can result from high altitude, strenuous exercise, anesthesia without adequate oxygenation, or other factors), hemoglobin S becomes 50 times less soluble than normal. A vaso-occlusive crisis can result as the increasingly viscous molecule crystallizes, deforming the erythrocyte into a crescent, or sickle, shape (see *Vaso-occlusive crisis: A chronology*).

Because they're rigid, sickled cells block capillary blood flow (see *Sickled cells: A closer look*). Local tissue hypoxia, further deoxygenation, and even more sickling result. This cycle can change even tiny obstructions into large infarctions. A heavy concentration of sickled cells thickens the blood, slowing circulation. If the patient also suffers dehydration from vomiting, diarrhea, excessive sweating, or diuretic use, the blood becomes even thicker, worsening his condition.

Reoxygenation usually turns sickled cells back into their normal shape. However, in some cases, the cell membrane suffers damage and the RBC remains permanently deformed. Constant formation and destruction of these cells leads to severe hemolytic anemia. Acidosis, an increased 2,3-diphosphoglycerate level, and a high MCHC can promote sickling.

Sickling crises, which can be preceded by viral or bacterial infection, may appear suddenly in any body region (most commonly in the chest, abdomen, and joints). The cumulative effect of sickling crises may cause the following damage:

- neurologic—hemiplegia (most common complication)
- ocular—retinal infarcts, vascular disease, and retinal detachment

Erythrocyte Disorders

Vaso-occlusive crisis: A chronology

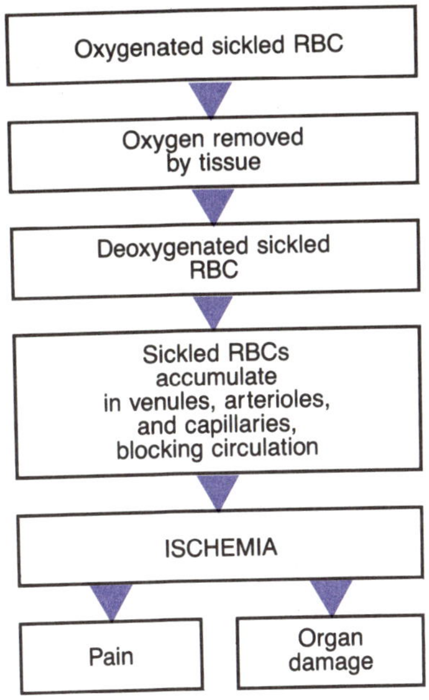

Sickled cells: A closer look

Containing hemoglobin S, an abnormal hemoglobin form, sickled RBCs become distorted and fragile.

As these cells aggregate and obstruct blood vessels, a painful sickle-cell crisis may occur.

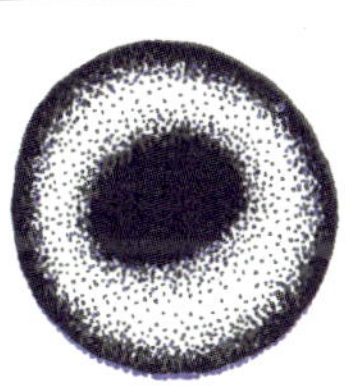

Normal red blood cell

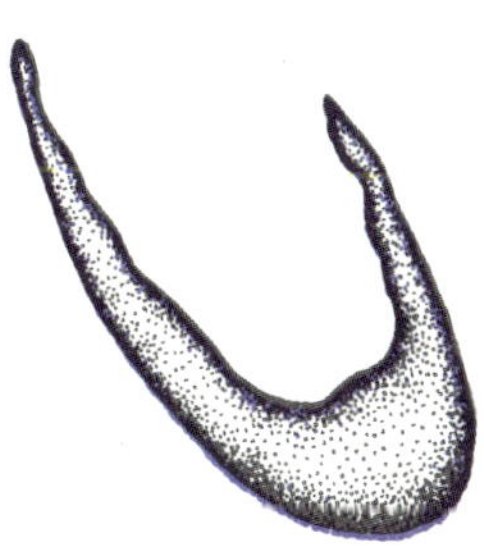

Sickled cell

- cardiopulmonary—impaired pulmonary function, hypoxemia from intrapulmonary arteriovenous shunting, and congestive heart failure from chronic severe anemia and hypoxemia
- GI—gallstone development from chronic hemolysis
- genitourinary—hematuria (painless but prolonged)
- integumentary—chronic lesions, particularly in severe cases, and jaundice
- skeletal—biconcave fish mouth vertebrae, aseptic necrosis of the femoral head, and osteomyelitis (commonly resulting from *Salmonella* infection).

Besides the painful vaso-occlusive crisis, sickle cell anemia can also cause:

- *aplastic (megaloblastic) crisis,* from bone marrow depression. Commonly associated with infection (usually viral), this crisis causes markedly decreased bone marrow activity and RBC hemolysis.
- *acute sequestration crisis.* Although rare, this crisis can occur in children aged 8 to 24 months. It may cause sudden RBC entrapment in the liver and spleen and, unless treated, can progress to hypovolemic shock and death.
- *hemolytic crisis.* Also rare, this usually affects sickle-cell anemia patients who have glucose-6-phosphate dehydrogenase deficiency, probably as a result of such complications as infection. Liver congestion and hepatomegaly typically occur from degenerative changes.

Sickle-cell anemia also causes long-term complications. Retinopathy and nephropathy, from organ infarction, are common. Premature death usually stems from infection or repeated small blood vessel occlusion and resultant major organ infarction or necrosis. For example, cerebral blood vessel occlusion can cause a cerebrovascular accident. Half of all sickle-cell anemia patients die by their early twenties; few live to middle age.

Individuals who inherit the abnormal gene from only one parent have the sickle-cell *trait*—a condition affecting about 8% of black Americans whose RBCs contain both normal hemoglobin and hemoglobin S molecules. These individuals experience sickling crises only when severe hypoxia develops. However, many have impaired urine-concentrating ability and some have recurrent episodes of painless hematuria stemming from renal medullary infarction. (For more information on this condition, see *Sickle-cell trait,* page 58.)

Assessment. The child with sickle-cell anemia typically suffers retarded growth and development, failure to thrive, and an increased risk of serious infection. Also expect delayed puberty (however, impaired fertility occurs rarely). During early childhood, palpation may reveal splenomegaly; but, as the child grows, the spleen shrinks. An adult with the disease may have narrow shoulders and hips, long arms and legs, a curved spine, a barrel chest, and an elongated skull.

Suspect a vaso-occlusive, aplastic, acute sequestration, or hemolytic crisis in a sickle-cell anemia patient who has pale lips, tongue, palms, or nail beds; who has a temperature above 104° F. (40° C.), or a fever of 100° F. (37.8° C.) or higher that persists for 2 days;

Continued on page 58

Erythrocyte Disorders

Sickle-cell trait

This relatively benign condition results from heterozygous inheritance of the abnormal hemoglobin S–producing gene. Like sickle-cell anemia, this condition is most common in blacks. Sickle-cell trait *never* progresses to sickle-cell anemia.

In persons with sickle-cell trait (also called carriers), 20% to 40% of their total hemoglobin is hemoglobin S; the remainder is normal.

Such persons usually have no symptoms. They have normal hemoglobin and hematocrit values and can expect a normal life span. Nevertheless, they must avoid situations that provoke hypoxia, since these occasionally cause a sickling crisis similar to that in sickle-cell anemia.

Genetic counseling is essential for sickle-cell carriers. If two sickle-cell carriers marry, each of their children has a 25% chance of inheriting sickle-cell anemia.

Hemolytic anemias—*continued*

or who complains of lethargy, listlessness, sleepiness, difficulty awakening, irritability, and severe pain.

Diagnostic tests that help confirm sickle-cell anemia include a stained blood smear revealing sickled cells and hemoglobin electrophoresis showing the hemoglobin S molecule. Ideally, electrophoresis should test umbilical cord blood samples from any infant whose parents are known sickle-cell trait carriers.

Additional laboratory studies typically reveal a below-normal RBC count, elevated WBC and platelet counts, a decreased erythrocyte sedimentation rate, an increased serum iron level, decreased RBC survival time, and reticulocytosis. Hemoglobin concentration levels may be subnormal or normal.

Intervention. Because sickle-cell anemia can't be cured, the doctor will order supportive symptomatic treatment. As ordered, give antibiotics and take measures to treat or prevent infection. In some cases, the doctor may order blood transfusions. (See *Preparing for a blood transfusion; Blood component therapy,* page 60; and *Recognizing transfusion reactions,* page 61.) Because the sickle-cell anemia patient needs extra folic acid, provide folic acid supplements, as ordered.

The doctor will treat painful crises promptly with analgesics and hydration. Early treatment may *prevent* a crisis, so he may give the patient a supply of analgesics. Between crises, the patient usually tolerates his disorder fairly well.

Nursing intervention. During a sickle-cell anemia crisis, apply warm compresses to painful areas and cover the patient with a blanket (cold compresses exacerbate the condition). Administer an analgesic-antipyretic, such as aspirin or acetaminophen, as ordered. When cultures indicate their need, give antibiotics as ordered. Encourage bed rest and place the patient in a sitting position.

During remission, help your patient avoid exacerbating his condition by:

- advising him to avoid tight clothing that restricts circulation
- warning him about conditions that provoke hypoxia—for example, strenuous exercise, vasoconstricting medications, cold temperatures (such as from swimming or drinking large amounts of ice water), unpressurized aircraft trips, and high altitudes
- stressing the importance of normal childhood immunizations, meticulous wound care, good oral hygiene, regular dental checkups, and a balanced diet to prevent infection
- emphasizing the need for prompt treatment of infection
- advising him to increase his fluid intake to prevent the dehydration that results from an impaired ability to concentrate urine properly. Parents should encourage a child with sickle-cell anemia to drink more fluids, especially in the summer, by offering pleasant-tasting drinks and ice pops.

To encourage normal development, warn parents against being overprotective. Although the child must avoid strenuous exercise, he can enjoy most everyday activities.

Erythrocyte Disorders

Teach the patient with sickle-cell trait about his condition and his ability to pass the trait or the anemia to his offspring. Suggest that parents of children with sickle-cell anemia consult a genetic counselor to learn about the risks for future offspring. These parents may also need psychological counseling to cope with guilt feelings. An appropriate community support group may prove helpful. Also recommend screening for other family members to determine whether they're heterozygous sickle-cell anemia carriers.

Sickle-cell anemia calls for special precautions during pregnancy. Warn a woman with sickle-cell anemia that she's a poor obstetric risk. Because oral contraceptives also pose a risk to such a patient,

Continued on page 60

Preparing for a blood transfusion

Before administration of a blood transfusion, the patient and blood component must be identified properly by two health care professionals. The following steps will ensure correct identification of the patient:

- Check the doctor's written order. Make sure you have the correct blood component in hand. Compare donor numbers and the ABO group on the transfusion record with the information on the blood component (see chart). If you're administering a blood component containing RBCs, also compare the Rh type.
- At the bedside, identify the patient as you would before obtaining a blood sample for pretransfusion testing. Make sure you check the full name and identification number on his wristband. Then ask the patient to state his name. If he can't respond, someone who knows him should identify him.
- Compare the full name and identification number on the patient's wristband with the name and number on the form attached to the blood component. Don't transfuse the blood if the information on the wristband doesn't correspond exactly with that on the blood component.
- Check the expiration date and time on the blood component. If an exact time isn't given, the component expires at midnight on the expiration date. A blood component should not be transfused after the expiration date and time. However, a transfusion that's already in progress may be completed after that time.
- If you discover a discrepancy during any of the above steps, postpone the transfusion until the discrepancy is resolved.
- Once you've determined that everything is in order, sign the transfusion record so that others will know who identified the patient and blood component. (The second health care professional involved in the identification process should cosign the record.)
- Make sure the label remains attached to the blood component until the transfusion is over.

ABO Compatibility

Patient's blood group	Antibodies present in plasma	Compatible RBCs	Compatible plasma
O	Anti-A and Anti-B	O	O, A, B, AB
A	Anti-B	A, O	A, AB
B	Anti-A	B, O	B, AB
AB	Neither Anti-A nor Anti-B	AB, A, B, O	AB

Donor's blood group	Antibodies present in plasma	Recipients compatible with donor RBCs	Recipients compatible with donor plasma
O	Anti-A and Anti-B	O, A, B, AB	O
A	Anti-B	A, AB	A, O
B	Anti-A	B, AB	B, O
AB	Neither Anti-A nor Anti-B	AB	AB, A, B, O

Rh Compatibility

Patient's Rh type	RBC Rh type for transfusion	Plasma Rh type for transfusion*
Positive	Positive or negative	Positive or negative
Negative	Negative	Positive or negative

*Rh antibodies are not normally present in plasma.

Erythrocyte Disorders

Hemolytic anemias—*continued*

refer her for birth control counseling by a gynecologist. If she becomes pregnant, encourage her to see an obstetrician, who will probably advise her to maintain a balanced diet during pregnancy and suggest that she take a folic acid supplement.

During surgery involving general anesthesia, a sickle-cell anemia patient requires adequate ventilation to prevent hypoxia. Make sure the surgeon and the anesthesiologist know that the patient has sickle-cell anemia. As needed and ordered, transfuse packed RBCs preoperatively.

Continued on page 62

Blood component therapy

All blood component products are extracted from whole blood, but each has different characteristics. So some blood components treat certain hematologic disorders better than others. The doctor will choose a blood component product based on how well it will treat your patient's condition. For example, if your patient needs volume replenishment quickly, he'll receive a volume expander. If his blood isn't clotting properly, he'll receive a product with clotting factors.

Here's a chart to help you learn more about blood component products and their uses.

Type	Uses	Nursing considerations
Whole blood RBCs, WBCs, platelets, plasma, and plasma clotting factors	• To restore blood volume and to replenish oxygen-carrying capacity in a patient with massive hemorrhage	• Administer through a large-gauge I.V. over 2 to 4 hours or as ordered.
Packed cells RBCs and 20% plasma; less sodium and potassium than in whole blood	• To replenish blood's oxygen-carrying capacity while minimizing risk of fluid overload in patients with severe anemia, slow blood loss, or congestive heart failure	Administer more slowly than whole blood (unless diluted with saline solution).
Washed cells RBCs and 20% plasma; fewer WBCs and platelets than in packed cells	• To replenish blood's oxygen-carrying capacity in patients previously sensitized by transfusions	• Administer at a slower rate than whole blood (unless diluted with saline solution).
Granulocytes WBCs and 20% plasma	• To treat life-threatening granulocytopenia ($<500/mm^3$)	• Administer rapidly. • Expect the patient to develop fever, chills, hypertension, or disorientation during transfusion; these are considered to be transfusion reactions.
Plasma (fresh frozen) Clotting Factors II, III, V, VII, IX, X, and XIII; fibrinogen; prothrombin; albumin; and globulins	• To treat patients with clotting factor deficiencies (the only treatment for Factor V deficiency) • To expand volume	• Fresh frozen plasma takes 20 minutes to thaw, so call the blood bank ahead of time. • Administer 1 unit over 1 hour.
Platelets Platelets, WBCs, and plasma	• To correct low platelet counts ($<10,000/mm^3$)	• Administer 1 unit over 10 minutes.
Cryoprecipitate Factors VIII and XIII and fibrinogen	• To replace clotting factors in patients with disseminated intravascular coagulation, hemophilia A, von Willebrand's disease, fibrinogen deficiency, or Factor XIII deficiency	• Administer rapidly *immediately after thawing,* to ensure factor activation.
Albumin (5% and 25%) 5% and 25% albumin from plasma	• To replace volume in patients suffering from shock, burns, hypoproteinemia, or hypoalbuminemia	• Administer 1 ml/minute or, *if the patient's in shock,* administer rapidly. • May administer with dextrose 5% in water.
Plasma protein fraction 5% albumin and globulin solution in saline solution	• To expand volume in patients with burns, hemorrhage, or hypoproteinemia	• Administer 1 ml/minute. • Risk of hepatitis or sensitization is low.
Prothrombin Factors II, VII, IX, and X	• To replace clotting factors in patients with hemophilia B or bleeding secondary to severe liver disease	• Prothrombin is used infrequently because of increased hepatitis risk.

Erythrocyte Disorders

Recognizing transfusion reactions

During a blood transfusion, your patient's at risk for developing any of five types of reactions. To learn to recognize them and to intervene appropriately, study this chart.

If your patient develops any sign or symptom of a reaction, immediately follow this procedure:
- Stop the transfusion.
- Change the I.V. tubing to prevent infusing any more blood. Save the tubing and blood bag for analysis.
- Administer saline solution I.V. to keep the vein open.
- Monitor the patient's vital signs at least every 15 minutes, depending on the patient's condition.
- Notify the doctor.
- Obtain urine and blood samples from the patient and send them to the laboratory. Return unused blood to the blood bank.
- Document the patient's reaction, noting the time the transfusion started and stopped, the amount of blood transfused, the patient's signs and symptoms, and all interventions.

Signs and symptoms	Nursing considerations
HEMOLYTIC REACTION	
Include chills, fever, low back pain, headache, chest pain, tachycardia, dyspnea, hypotension, nausea and vomiting, restlessness, anxiety, shock	• Expect to place the patient in a supine position, with his legs elevated 20° to 30°, and to administer oxygen, fluids, and epinephrine to correct shock. • Expect to administer mannitol to maintain the patient's renal circulation. • Expect to insert an indwelling (Foley) catheter to monitor the patient's urinary output (should be about 100 ml/hr). • Expect to administer antipyretics to lower the patient's fever. If his fever persists, expect to apply a hypothermia blanket or to give tepid sponge or alcohol baths.
PLASMA PROTEIN INCOMPATIBILITY	
Include chills, fever, flushing, abdominal pain, diarrhea, dyspnea, hypotension	• Expect to place the patient in a supine position, with his legs elevated 20° to 30°, and to administer oxygen, fluids, and epinephrine to correct shock. • Expect to administer corticosteroids.
BLOOD CONTAMINATION	
Include chills, fever, abdominal pain, nausea and vomiting, bloody diarrhea, hypotension	• Expect to administer fluids, antibiotics, corticosteroids, vasopressors, and a fresh transfusion.
FEBRILE REACTION	
Range from mild chills, flushing, and fever to extreme signs and symptoms resembling a hemolytic reaction	• Expect to administer an antipyretic and an antihistamine for a *mild* reaction. Expect to treat a *severe* reaction the same as a hemolytic reaction.
ALLERGIC REACTION	
Range from pruritus, urticaria, hives, facial swelling, chills, fever, nausea and vomiting, headache, and wheezing to laryngeal edema, respiratory distress, and shock	• If the patient's only sign of reaction is hives, expect to restart the infusion, as ordered, at a slower rate. • Expect to administer parenteral antihistamines or, for a severe reaction, epinephrine or corticosteroids.

Erythrocyte Disorders

Hemolytic anemias—*continued*

A man with sickle-cell anemia may develop sudden, painful episodes of priapism. Reassure him that these episodes are common and have no permanent harmful effects.

Thalassemias
Like sickle-cell anemia, thalassemias are inherited hemoglobin synthesis disorders. A mixed and complex group, they involve absent or diminished synthesis of one of hemoglobin A's globin chains.

Two pairs of polypeptide chains—alpha chains and beta chains—make up hemoglobin. In thalassemias, diminished synthesis can affect either pair. Structurally, the chains are normal but the genetic defect decreases their number. In *alpha-thalassemia,* alpha chain synthesis slows; in *beta-thalassemia,* beta chain synthesis slows. Some patients with beta-thalassemia have no normal hemoglobin, only hemoglobin S and the minor hemoglobins.

In the most severe alpha-thalassemia form—hydrops fetalis—severe anemia and congestive heart failure effects render fetuses hydropic. These fetuses are stillborn or die shortly after birth. Prenatal diagnosis can detect the condition.

Beta-thalassemia (by far, the most common thalassemia) occurs in three clinical forms: thalassemia major, intermedia, and minor. The severity of the resulting anemia depends on whether the patient's homozygous or heterozygous for the thalassemic trait. Prognosis for beta-thalassemia varies. Patients with thalassemia major seldom survive to adulthood; children with thalassemia intermedia develop normally into adulthood, although puberty's usually delayed; persons with thalassemia minor can expect a normal life span.

Assessment. Signs and symptoms of thalassemia major include jaundice, cholelithiasis, leg ulcers, and spleen enlargement. The disease can be detected soon after birth, with typical erythrocyte changes sometimes identifiable by age 6 weeks. Other signs include poor growth and development (from chronic anemia) and changes in the skull, long bones, and hands (from ineffective marrow erythroid hyperplasia). Children commonly suffer recurrent infections. Iron deposits from blood transfusions and accelerated iron uptake and deposition in parenchymal tissue cause hemosiderosis. Myocardial siderosis causes conduction defects and heart failure—the overwhelming cause of death in affected children.

Ineffective erythropoiesis leads to erythroid hyperplasia, causing severe medullary expansion and bone remodeling. Marrow hyperplasia and facial bone expansion cause prominent cheekbones, which obscure the nasal base and expose the upper teeth. Extension extramedullary erythropoiesis results in severe hepatosplenomegaly; accelerated bilirubin production commonly leads to biliary tract disease.

In thalassemia major, laboratory results show lowered RBC and hemoglobin levels and elevated reticulocyte, bilirubin, and urinary and fecal urobilinogen levels. A low serum folate level indicates increased folate utilization by the hypertrophied bone marrow. A peripheral blood smear reveals target cells (extremely thin and fragile RBCs), pale nucleated RBCs, and marked anisocytosis. Skull

Erythrocyte Disorders

Thalassemia major

This illustration of an X-ray shows a characteristic skull abnormality in thalassemia major: diploetic fibers extending perpendicularly from internal laminae, resembling hair standing on end.

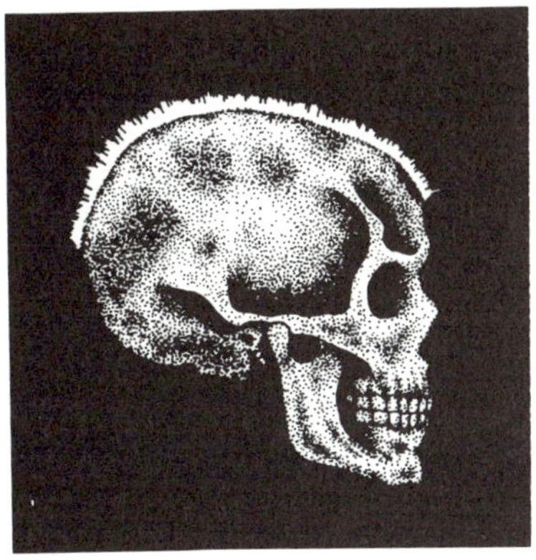

and long-bone X-rays show thinning and widening of the marrow space from overactive bone marrow. Skull and vertebral bones may appear granular; long bones may show osteoporotic areas. The phalanges may also be deformed (rectangular or biconvex). Hemoglobin electrophoresis demonstrates a significant Hb F rise and a slight Hb A_2 increase. Diagnosis must rule out iron-deficiency anemia, which also produces hypochromia and microcytic RBCs.

In thalassemia intermedia, laboratory results show hypochromia and microcytic RBCs, but the anemia's less severe than that in thalassemia major. In thalassemia minor, laboratory results show hypochromia and microcytic RBCs. Hemoglobin electrophoresis shows a significant Hb A_2 increase and a moderate Hb F rise.

Intervention. Treatment of thalassemia major is essentially supportive. For example, infections require prompt treatment with appropriate antibiotics. Folic acid supplements help maintain folic acid levels despite increased requirements. Packed RBC transfusions raise hemoglobin levels but must be used judiciously to minimize iron overload. Splenectomy and bone marrow transplantation have been tried, but their effectiveness has not been confirmed.

Thalassemia intermedia and thalassemia minor generally don't require treatment.

Iron supplements are contraindicated in all thalassemia forms.

Treatment of children proves more difficult. Regular blood transfusions may minimize retarded physical and mental development, but transfusions increase the risk of deadly hemosiderosis and iron overload. Continuous subcutaneous infusion of iron-chelating agents has recently proved effective in producing a negative overall iron balance. The doctor may perform splenectomy if rapid splenic sequestration of transfused RBCs necessitates more transfusions.

Nursing intervention. Care for the thalassemia patient as you would for any anemia patient. Watch for adverse reactions—shaking chills, fever, rash, pruritus, urticaria—during and after transfusions. Teach parents to watch for signs of hepatitis and iron overload—always possible with frequent transfusions.

Stress the importance of good nutrition, meticulous wound care, periodic dental checkups, and other measures to prevent infection.

Provide emotional support to help the patient and his family cope with the chronic nature of the illness and the need for lifelong transfusions. Discuss with the parents of a young patient various options for healthy physical and creative outlets. Such a child must avoid strenuous athletic activity because of increased oxygen demand and the tendency toward pathologic fractures, but he may participate in less stressful activities.

If parents have questions about the susceptibility of future offspring, refer them for genetic counseling. Also refer adult patients with thalassemia minor or thalassemia intermedia for genetic counseling. They need to recognize the risk of transmitting thalassemia major to their children if they marry another person with thalassemia.

Continued on page 64

Erythrocyte Disorders

Hemolytic anemias—*continued*

If such persons choose to marry and have children, all their children should undergo evaluation for thalassemia by age 1. Be sure to tell persons with thalassemia minor that the condition's benign.

Polycythemias

In these disorders, which include polycythemia vera, spurious polycythemia, and secondary polycythemia, RBC production increases abnormally. Polycythemias may arise secondary to cardiac or pulmonary disease or prolonged exposure to high altitudes, or they may be idiopathic.

Polycythemia vera
Also known as primary polycythemia, erythremia, polycythemia rubra vera, splenomegalic polycythemia, and Vaquez-Osler disease, this polycythemia form is chronic and myeloproliferative. Besides increased RBC mass, it's characterized by leukocytosis, thrombocytosis, and increased hemoglobin concentration levels, with normal or decreased plasma volume. Uncontrolled and rapid cellular reproduction and maturation cause proliferation or hyperplasia of all bone marrow cells (panmyelosis). The cause of such uncontrolled cellular activity remains unknown but may be a pluripotent stem cell defect.

Polycythemia vera usually strikes persons aged 40 to 60, most commonly men of Jewish ancestry. It rarely affects children or blacks and doesn't seem to be familial. Prognosis depends on age at diagnosis, treatment used, and complications. Untreated polycythemia vera, especially when accompanied by myeloid metaplasia, carries a high mortality.

Assessment. In its early stages, polycythemia vera usually remains asymptomatic (increased hematocrit level may be an incidental finding). However, as altered circulation secondary to increased RBC mass leads to hypervolemia and hyperviscosity, the patient may complain of a vague feeling of fullness in the head, dizziness, headache, tinnitus, visual disturbances, and other symptoms, depending on the body system affected. (See *Polycythemia vera: Recognizing clinical features.*)

Paradoxically, hemorrhage can arise as a complication of polycythemia vera caused by defective platelet function or by hyperviscosity and local effects of excess RBCs exerting pressure on distended venous and capillary walls. The patient may complain of bruising with epistaxis and gingival bleeding.

Laboratory studies confirm polycythemia vera by showing increased RBC mass and normal arterial oxygen saturation along with splenomegaly or at least two of the following:
- thrombocytosis
- leukocytosis
- elevated leukocyte alkaline phosphatase level
- elevated serum vitamin B_{12} or unbound B_{12}-binding capacity.

Patients typically show increased uric acid production, leading to hyperuricemia and hyperuricuria. Other laboratory results include an increased blood histamine level, a below-normal serum iron level,

Erythrocyte Disorders

Polycythemia vera: Recognizing clinical features

Body system	Findings	Causes
Neurologic	Headache or full sensation in head, lethargy, syncope, tinnitus, paresthesia, impaired mental function	Hypervolemia and hyperviscosity from congested vessels, increased oxyhemoglobin level, and reduced hemoglobin level
Eye, ear, nose, and throat	Visual disturbances (blurring, diplopia, scotoma, engorged fundal and retinal veins) and congestion of conjunctiva, retina, retinal veins, and oral mucous membrane	Hypervolemia, hyperviscosity
	Epistaxis, gingival bleeding	Capillary bed engorgement
Respiratory	Dyspnea, lung congestion	Hypervolemia, hyperviscosity
Cardiovascular	Hypertension, tachycardia	Hypervolemia, hyperviscosity
	Intermittent claudication, thrombosis and embolism, angina, thrombophlebitis	Hypervolemia, thrombocytosis, vascular disease
	Hemorrhage	Capillary bed engorgement
Gastrointestinal	Epigastric distress	Hypervolemia, hyperviscosity
	Early satiety and fullness	Hepatosplenomegaly
	Peptic ulcer pain	Gastric thrombosis and hemorrhage
	Enlarged liver and spleen	Congestion, extramedullary hematopoiesis, myeloid metaplasia
	Weight loss	Hypermetabolism
Integumentary	Pruritus (especially after a hot bath)	Basophilia (secondary to histamine release)
	Urticaria	Altered histamine metabolism
	Plethora (especially of the face, ears, nose, lips, and distal arm and leg regions)	Hypervolemia, hyperviscosity
	Ecchymosis	Hemorrhage
	Night sweats	Hypermetabolism
Musculoskeletal	Swollen, painful joints	Increased urate production

and decreased or absent urinary erythropoietin. Bone marrow biopsy reveals panmyelosis.

Planning. Focus your nursing care on preventing complications, providing comfort measures, and encouraging patient independence.

Nursing diagnoses. Before determining your nursing care plan, develop the nursing diagnosis by identifying the patient's actual or potential problem, then relating it to its cause. Possible nursing diagnoses for a patient with polycythemia vera include:

- activity intolerance; related to immobility from painful, swollen joints and dyspnea
- nutrition, alteration in (less than body requirements); related to fatigue and weakness
- self-concept (disturbance in body image); related to plethora
- mobility, impaired physical; related to painful joints

Continued on page 66

Erythrocyte Disorders

Polycythemias—*continued*

- skin integrity, impairment of (potential); related to plethora and pruritus
- cardiac output, alteration in (decreased); related to hypervolemia and hyperviscosity
- comfort, alteration in (pain); related to swollen joints.

Intervention. Phlebotomy, the primary treatment, rapidly reduces RBC mass. The frequency of phlebotomy and the amount of blood removed each time depends on the patient's condition. The patient can usually withstand a 350- to 500-ml blood loss every other day until his hematocrit level falls to the low-normal range. After repeated phlebotomies, he develops iron deficiency, which stabilizes RBC production, making phlebotomy less necessary.

Phlebotomy doesn't reduce WBC or platelet count and won't control the hyperuricemia that appears with bone marrow cell proliferation. In severe cases, myelosuppressive therapy may help. Radioactive phosphorus (^{32}P) or chemotherapeutic agents, such as melphalan, busulfan, or cyclophosphamide, usually control the disease satisfactorily. However, because these agents may cause leukemia, the doctor will order them only for elderly patients and those with serious problems that phlebotomy can't control. Patients of any age who've had previous thrombotic problems may need myelosuppressive therapy.

Nursing intervention. For the patient with polycythemia vera, you'll need to perform the following interventions:

- Tell the patient to watch for and report any symptoms of iron deficiency (such as pallor, weight loss, asthenia, and glossitis).
- Keep the patient active and ambulatory to prevent thrombosis. If bed rest proves necessary, encourage a daily program of both active and passive range-of-motion exercises.
- Watch for such complications as hypervolemia, thrombocytosis, and signs of an impending cerebrovascular accident (decreased sensation, numbness, transitory paralysis, fleeting blindness, headache, and epistaxis).
- Instruct the patient to guard against injury and to use caution in daily activities. Advise him to avoid iron-rich foods and to eat small meals to help control GI bleeding.

Sample nursing care plan: Polycythemia vera

Nursing diagnosis	**Expected outcomes**
Activity intolerance; related to immobility from painful, swollen joints and dyspnea	The patient will: • explain the reason for his activity intolerance. • demonstrate increased activity and energy. • function at his highest activity level.
Nursing interventions	**Discharge planning**
• Instruct patient to alternate rest and activity periods. • Encourage patient to eat small, frequent meals to help him gain strength. • Advise patient to avoid hot showers and baths. • Teach patient to elevate the painful joint on pillows. • Evaluate the effectiveness of pain medication.	• Teach patient techniques to conserve energy and improve activity level at home and at work. • Consult community health nurse about follow-up care in patient's home, as needed. • Review with patient the action, use, dosage, and adverse effects of his medications. • Remind patient to keep follow-up appointments, as needed.

Erythrocyte Disorders

- Regularly examine the patient closely for signs of bleeding. Teach him about the most common bleeding sites (the nose, gingiva, and skin) so that he can check for bleeding himself. Advise him to report any abnormal bleeding promptly.
- To compensate for increased uric acid production, give the patient additional fluids, administer allopurinol as ordered, and alkalinize the urine to prevent uric acid calculi.
- If the patient has symptomatic splenomegaly, suggest or provide small, frequent meals followed by a rest period to prevent nausea and vomiting.
- Report acute abdominal pain immediately; it may signal splenic infarction, renal calculi, or abdominal organ thrombosis.
- Provide rest periods and adequate nutrition to relieve fatigue.
- Administer antihistamines such as Benadryl, antipruritic lotions, or medicated baths, as ordered, to relieve pruritus.

If the patient requires phlebotomy:
- Explain the procedure and reassure the patient that it will relieve distressing symptoms. Check blood pressure, pulse rate, and respirations. During phlebotomy, make sure he's lying down comfortably to prevent vertigo and syncope. Stay alert for tachycardia, clamminess, or complaints of vertigo. If these reactions occur, stop the procedure.
- Immediately after phlebotomy, check the patient's blood pressure and pulse rate. To prevent a vasovagal attack or orthostatic hypotension, have him sit up for about 5 minutes before allowing him to walk. Also have him drink 24 oz (700 ml) of juice or water.

If the patient's receiving myelosuppressive chemotherapy:
- Monitor CBC and platelet count before and during therapy. If leukopenia develops in an outpatient, warn him that he has low infection resistance. Advise him to avoid crowds and make sure he knows how to recognize infection symptoms. If leukopenia develops in a hospitalized patient who needs reverse isolation, follow your hospital's guidelines.
- Teach the patient about possible adverse reactions (nausea, vomiting, and susceptibility to infection) that may follow alkylating agent administration. Alopecia usually occurs after use of busulfan and cyclophosphamide. Sterile hemorrhagic cystitis may follow cyclophosphamide use (however, forcing fluids can prevent this effect). Watch for and report all adverse reactions. If nausea and vomiting occur, begin antiemetic therapy, as ordered, and adjust the patient's diet.

If your patient's receiving ^{32}P treatment:
- Explain the procedure to relieve anxiety. Tell the patient that he may require repeated phlebotomies until ^{32}P takes effect. Make sure you have a blood sample for baseline CBC and platelet count measurement before treatment begins.
- To facilitate the procedure and prevent extravasation, have the patient lie down during I.V. ^{32}P administration. He should remain prone for 15 to 20 minutes after the procedure.

Evaluation. Base your evaluation on the expected outcomes listed on the nursing care plan. To determine whether your patient's improved, ask yourself the following questions:

Continued on page 68

Erythrocyte Disorders

Polycythemias—*continued*

- Can the patient tell you why his activity is limited?
- Is his activity level increasing? Does he have more energy?
- Is he functioning at his highest activity level?

The answers to these questions will help you evaluate your patient's status and the effectiveness of his care. Keep in mind that these questions stem from the sample care plan on page 66. Your questions may differ.

Spurious polycythemia
An increased hematocrit level and a normal or below-normal RBC total mass characterize this disorder. Also known as relative polycythemia, stress erythrocytosis, stress polycythemia, benign polycythemia, Gaisböck's syndrome, and pseudopolycythemia, spurious polycythemia results from decreased plasma volume and subsequent hemoconcentration. Usually affecting middle-aged persons, it occurs more commonly in men than in women.

Spurious polycythemia can arise in the following circumstances:
- *dehydration.* Conditions that promote severe fluid loss decrease plasma levels, leading to hemoconcentration. Such conditions include persistent vomiting or diarrhea, burns, adrenocortical insufficiency, aggressive diuretic therapy, decreased fluid intake, diabetic acidosis, and renal disease.
- *stress-induced hemoconcentration.* Stress can lead to hemoconcentration by an unknown mechanism (possibly by temporarily decreasing circulating plasma volume or causing vascular erythrocyte redistribution). Erythrocytosis with a chronically elevated hematocrit level is particularly common in the middle-aged man who smokes and has a type A (tense, hard-driving, anxious) personality.
- *high-normal RBC mass and low-normal plasma volume level.* In many patients, an increased hematocrit level merely reflects a normally high RBC mass and low plasma volume. This especially occurs among nonsmoking, nonobese patients with no history of hypertension.

Other factors that may contribute to spurious polycythemia include hypertension, thromboembolitic disease, elevated serum cholesterol and uric acid levels, and a familial tendency.

Assessment. Spurious polycythemia usually causes no specific symptoms. The patient may complain of such vague problems as headache, dizziness, and fatigue. Less commonly, diaphoresis, dyspnea, and claudication may develop.

Typically, the patient has a ruddy appearance, a short neck, slight hypertension, and a tendency to hypoventilate when recumbent. He shows no associated hepatosplenomegaly but may have cardiac or pulmonary disease.

Expect elevated hemoglobin, hematocrit, and RBC levels and normal RBC mass, arterial oxygen saturation, and bone marrow results. Plasma volume may be below-normal or normal. Other laboratory studies may reveal hypercholesterolemia, hyperlipemia, or hyperuricemia. Spurious polycythemia can be distinguished from true polycythemia vera by its characteristic normal RBC mass, elevated hematocrit level, and absent leukocytosis.

Erythrocyte Disorders

Intervention. Treatment aims to correct dehydration and prevent life-threatening thromboembolism. Rehydration with appropriate fluids and electrolytes forms the primary therapy for spurious polycythemia secondary to dehydration. Therapy must also include appropriate measures to prevent continuing fluid loss.

Nursing intervention. During rehydration, carefully monitor the patient's fluid intake and output to maintain fluid and electrolyte balance. To prevent thromboembolism in a predisposed patient, suggest regular exercise and a low-cholesterol diet. Antilipemic agents may also be necessary. The obese patient may need a low-calorie diet.

Thoroughly explain spurious polycythemia, all diagnostic measures, and therapy. Expect the hard-driving patient who's predisposed to this disease to be more inquisitive and anxious than the average patient. Answer his questions honestly and reassure him that he can control symptoms by complying with treatment.

Whenever appropriate, suggest counseling about the patient's work habits and lack of relaxation. If the patient smokes, make sure he understands the importance of quitting. Refer him to an antismoking program, if necessary.

Emphasize the need for follow-up examinations every 3 to 4 months after leaving the hospital.

Secondary polycythemia
Also known as reactive polycythemia, secondary polycythemia involves excessive production of circulating erythrocytes. It may stem from hypoxia, tumor, or disease. The disease occurs most commonly in persons living at high altitudes.

Secondary polycythemia may result from increased production of erythropoietin, which stimulates bone marrow to increase erythrocyte production. Increased erythropoietin production may be a compensatory response to hypoxemia resulting from chronic obstructive pulmonary disease, hemoglobin abnormalities (such as carboxyhemoglobinemia, seen in heavy smokers), congestive heart failure (causing a decreased ventilation-perfusion ratio), right-to-left cardiac shunting (as in transposition of the great vessels), central or peripheral alveolar hypoventilation (as in barbiturate intoxication or pickwickian syndrome), and low oxygen content of air at high altitudes. When hypoxemia isn't the cause, secondary polycythemia may show up during treatment for an underlying disease.

Increased erythropoietin production may also occur in response to renal disease (such as renovascular impairment, cysts, or hydronephrosis), central nervous system disease (such as encephalitis and parkinsonism), neoplasms (such as renal tumors, uterine myomas, or cerebellar hemangiomas), or endocrine disorders (such as Cushing's syndrome, Bartter's syndrome, or pheochromocytomas). Rarely, secondary polycythemia results from a recessive genetic trait.

Assessment. In the hypoxic patient, suggestive physical findings include plethora, emphysema, and hypoxemia with hepatospleno-

Continued on page 70

Erythrocyte Disorders

Polycythemias—*continued*

megaly or hypertension. Clubbed fingers may occur with an underlying cardiovascular disease.

Suggestive laboratory findings include increased RBC mass, urinary erythropoietin, and blood histamine levels with below-normal or normal arterial oxygen saturation. Bone marrow biopsies reveal hyperplasia confined to the erythroid series. Unlike polycythemia vera, secondary polycythemia isn't accompanied by leukocytosis or thrombocytosis.

Intervention. Treatment aims to correct the underlying disease or environmental condition. In severe secondary polycythemia where high altitude contributes, the patient may need to relocate. If secondary polycythemia has produced hazardous hyperviscosity or if the patient doesn't respond to treatment for the primary disease, phlebotomy may be effective. The doctor will perform emergency phlebotomy to prevent impending vascular occlusion or before emergency surgery. Before surgery, expect him to remove excess erythrocytes and reinfuse the patient's plasma.

Because a polycythemia patient has an increased hemorrhage risk during and after surgery, he should avoid elective surgery until his condition has been controlled. Generally, secondary polycythemia disappears with correction of the primary disease.

Nursing interventions. Keep the patient as active as possible to decrease the thrombosis risk from increased blood viscosity. Reduce his calorie and sodium intake to counteract the tendency to hypertension.

Before and after phlebotomy, check his blood pressure when he's in a supine position. After the procedure, give him about 24 oz (700 ml) of water or juice to drink, as ordered. To prevent syncope, have him sit up for about 5 minutes before walking.

Emphasize the importance of regular blood studies—every 2 to 3 months—even after the disease is under control. Be sure to teach the patient and family about the underlying disorder.

Leukocyte Disorders: Acute and Chronic Leukemias

Janet N. Pavel, who wrote this chapter, is Chief Nurse in the Department of Transfusion Medicine, National Institutes of Health, Bethesda, Md. She received her ADN from Montgomery College, Rockville, Md.

Leukocytes, or white blood cells (WBCs), form the body's mobile defense system. Unlike erythrocytes (red blood cells), which remain in blood vessels, leukocytes perform their functions in body tissues, squeezing through intercellular spaces in the capillary wall.

An uncontrolled proliferation of leukocytes signals leukemia, the major leukocyte disorder. (For other causes, see *Elevated leukocyte levels: Identifying causes.*) This chapter discusses the four major leukemia forms. To better understand these diseases, first review some basic information about leukocytes by reading what follows.

Leukocyte appearance, types, and functions. Named for their lack of pigmentation, leukocytes appear white or colorless, depending on the refraction. Usually larger than erythrocytes, leukocytes have prominent nuclei. In a normal blood sample, they're greatly outnumbered by erythrocytes (by about 700 to 1).

Leukocytes lack uniform size, shape, and appearance. Studies have revealed six different leukocyte types:

- neutrophils
- eosinophils
- basophils
- monocytes
- lymphocytes
- plasma cells.

These types fall into two main categories—granulocytes and nongranulocytes. Granulocytes—neutrophils, eosinophils, and basophils—have granules in their cytoplasm. These cells carry out several essential defensive processes, including chemotaxis (movement toward or away from a chemical stimulus), phagocytosis (engulfment and digestion of harmful particles), and microbe destruction. (It's interesting to note that granulocytes produce myeloperoxidase, an enzyme that's responsible for the green color of pus.) Most granulocytes leave the blood randomly, regardless of age, when they're needed in the tissues. Only a few grow old in the blood and must be destroyed.

Neutrophils, the most abundant granulocytes, account for about 50% to 70% of all leukocytes. These phagocytic cells circulate briefly in the bloodstream, then enter tissues and body cavities where they migrate to sites of bacterial proliferation and inflammation. Myeloproliferative disorders, invasive tumors, and inflammation elevate the neutrophil count. Only mature neutrophils can carry out phagocytosis effectively. A slightly immature form, called a band neutrophil (or band), normally represents about 3% of leukocytes. In the diagnostic finding referred to as a "shift to the left," the number of bands and other immature neutrophils increases (cell production moves toward the left on the neutrophil maturation chart). This usually indicates a localized infection, such as appendicitis. The degree of shift reflects the infection's severity. In a "shift to the right," the number of mature neutrophils increases; this commonly occurs with vitamin B_{12} deficiency anemia. Both leftward and rightward shifts can occur in early stages of chronic myelocytic leukemia. Corticosteroid therapy increases the neutrophil count but decreases the number of mature, effective neutrophils. Consequently, corticosteroid use makes a person more susceptible to serious infection.

Continued on page 72

Elevated leukocyte levels: Identifying causes

Levels of certain leukocytes—indicated by the white blood cell differential count—typically rise with various diseases and conditions. For example, abnormally high eosinophil, basophil, lymphocyte, and monocyte levels commonly accompany leukemia. Below, we show some other causes of elevated leukocyte levels.

Neutrophils
Levels elevated by:
- Bacterial infections
- Inflammation
- Invasive tumors
- Stress

Eosinophils
Levels elevated by:
- Allergic disorders
- Drug reactions
- Parasitic infections
- Certain skin disorders
- Some cancers

Basophils
Levels elevated by:
- Asthma
- Blood disorders
- Chronic inflammation
- Some cancers

Monocytes
Levels elevated by:
- Chronic infections
- Liver disease

Lymphocytes
Levels elevated by:
- Viral infections
- Some cancers

Plasma cells
Levels elevated by:
- Plasma cell myeloma

Leukocyte Disorders

Continued

Eosinophils account for 2% to 4% of leukocytes. Prevalent in the intestinal mucosa and lungs, they protect the body against foreign proteins. Eosinophils carry out some phagocytosis, but researchers believe their main contribution lies in detoxifying foreign proteins. Proliferating during an allergic reaction, they migrate to the reaction site and remove the antigen-antibody complex from the blood when the immune response ends. They may also help eliminate blood clots by secreting plasmin, an enzyme involved in clot dissolution.

Basophils account for just 0.3% to 2% of all leukocytes. Nonphagocytic, they serve mainly to secrete histamine and heparin. They resemble mast cells—connective tissue cells, found near many capillaries, that release heparin into the blood. Basophils play a key role in anaphylaxis and other systemic allergic reactions, undergoing granulation and releasing heparin and histamine into the blood. They also help prevent blood clot formation and growth and speed lipid removal from the blood after a fatty meal.

Nongranulocytes, which lack cytoplasmic granules, include monocytes, lymphocytes, and plasma cells. *Monocytes,* representing about 3% to 8% of leukocytes, are immature phagocytic cells. When migrating to tissues and body cavities, they mature into macrophages, highly efficient phagocytes that consume invading organisms. The largest leukocytes, monocytes can ingest malarial parasites and entire erythrocytes and excel at phagocytizing necrotic tissue from chronic inflammation.

Present in all tissues, macrophages abound in filter organs, including the liver, spleen, lungs, and lymph nodes. *Free* macrophages wander from the blood through vascular endothelial membranes to trap material for phagocytosis. They collect at inflammation sites and in peritoneal, pleural, and synovial fluid. *Fixed* macrophages (such as histiocytes) remain in the liver, spleen, lungs, lymph nodes, bone marrow, and adrenal and pituitary glands. They engulf microorganisms and cellular and noncellular debris (such as silica dust).

Monocytes serve as the mobile units of the mononuclear phagocytic system (MPS), formerly known as the reticuloendothelial system; most MPS cells stay in the bone marrow, liver, and lymph nodes.

Lymphocytes, which make up about 25% to 30% of leukocytes, differentiate into B lymphocytes (B cells) and T lymphocytes (T cells) when mature. B cells differentiate into plasma cells, which, in turn, secrete immunoglobulins (antibodies). T cells carry out cell-mediated immune responses. (For more information on lymphocytes, see Chapter 7.)

Normally absent from the blood, *plasma cells* are found in the spleen and in lymphatic and connective tissue. They produce the most immunoglobulins. (For a more detailed discussion of plasma cells and related disorders, see Chapter 8.)

Leukopoiesis. This term refers to leukocyte production and development. All granulocytes and a few lymphocytes and monocytes derive from bone marrow. Most lymphocytes originate in lymphatic tissue. (Although the bone marrow contains many lymphocytes, most of these presumably have traveled there from the bloodstream after forming in lymphatic tissue.)

Granulocytosis

This diagnostic finding reflects elevated levels of granulocytes—especially neutrophils and their precursors (bands and, in some cases, metamyelocytes). A common finding, granulocytosis can be relative or absolute on the white blood cell differential.

Granulocytosis may arise from the following conditions:
- bacterial infection, particularly by pus-producing bacteria
- inflammation, such as with myositis and vasculitis
- tissue necrosis
- toxic conditions, such as acidosis, eclampsia, gout, and uremia
- other factors, such as acute hemorrhage or hemolysis (particularly in children) and splenectomy.

The bone marrow produces granulocytes as needed and can step up production when infection or stress occurs. With a peripheral bacterial invasion, for example, granulocytes migrate from the blood to the bacteria site. This migration accelerates the release of bone marrow reserves. Cell production in the marrow then increases to meet demand.

A leftward shift in the neutrophil count may accompany granulocytosis. This shift represents an increase in the ratio of nonsegmented (immature) neutrophils to segmented (mature) neutrophils. (The term *segmented* refers to sectioning of the mature cell's nucleus into two or more lobes.)

Assessment findings and intervention for granulocytosis depend on the underlying cause.

Leukocyte Disorders

Granulocytopenia

Marked by decreased levels of granulocytes (specifically neutrophils), granulocytopenia can result from decreased granulocyte production (caused, for example, by toxic agents), increased granulocyte destruction (from such conditions as hypersplenism), congenital defects (for example, Chédiak-Higashi syndrome), or infection. Untreated, granulocytopenia causes death in about 80% of patients. (*Note:* Leukopenia refers to depression of the *total* leukocyte count.)

Agranulocytosis—a neutrophil level below 300/µl—is the most severe form of granulocytopenia. This condition greatly increases the infection risk, because neutrophils account for about 55% to 75% of all leukocytes. Agranulocytosis may stem from use of certain drugs or exposure to toxic chemicals.

Assessment. Signs and symptoms of granulocytopenia include malaise, discomfort, lassitude, muscle ache, headache, sore throat, fever, tachycardia, and mouth ulcers. A white blood cell differential count confirms the disorder.

Intervention. The doctor will order treatment measures to correct the underlying disorder, possibly including antibiotics. Follow these guidelines when caring for the patient:
- Ease patient discomfort from fever and chills.
- Protect the patient from infection, for example, by washing your hands thoroughly and preventing him from exposure to infectious persons.
- Remove necrotic tissue from the patient's mouth by irrigating with warm saline solution.
- Monitor the patient's leukocyte count. If the count drops extremely low, notify the doctor immediately (he may order protective isolation).
- Encourage bed rest and provide a high-protein diet to help combat debilitation.
- As ordered, apply an ice collar and administer lozenges to help relieve severe throat pain.

The life span of leukocytes remains unknown. Some evidence suggests that granulocytes live three days, at most; other studies indicate that they live about 12 days. Some small lymphocytes apparently survive much longer—up to 200 days or more.

Leukopoiesis is controlled mainly by chemotaxis—movement in response to release of chemicals from dead or dying granulocytes and bacteria. Other controlling factors include infection, androgens, antibodies, and blood loss into body cavities.

Leukemia

Leukemia refers to the cancerous proliferation of one or more blood-forming cellular elements, usually leukocytes (however, erythroleukemia, an extremely rare leukemia, involves erythrocytes). Leukemia leads to functionally impaired, immature cells (blasts). These abnormal leukocytes circulate in peripheral blood and accumulate in the bone marrow, where they disrupt hematopoiesis. As a result, production of normal leukocytes, erythrocytes, and platelets decreases, leading to anemia, leukopenia, and thrombocytopenia—a triad collectively known as pancytopenia.

Leukemic cells proliferate mainly in the bone marrow; however, they may also infiltrate the spleen, lymph nodes, central nervous system (CNS), kidneys, skin, tonsils, and gingivae.

Although leukemia's precise cause remains unknown, research suggests that exposure to certain chemicals (such as benzene) or large doses of radiation plays a role. Other possible factors include viral infection, immunologic defects, and genetic abnormalities. Also, acute leukemias have a higher incidence among persons with certain congenital conditions, such as Down's syndrome.

Leukemia's pathogenesis also remains unclear. The most widely accepted theory holds that leukemic cells develop from a single cell mutation. The resulting clones survive longer and, despite reproducing more slowly, have longer reproductive lives than normal cells. However, they fail to mature and differentiate, thus producing few, if any, fully developed cells.

Leukemia occurs more frequently in adults; however, children usually have a better prognosis. Despite treatment advances, leukemia remains the second leading cause of death among children aged 4 to 14.

Leukemia types. Leukemia can be acute or chronic; myelocytic or lymphocytic. (See *How leukemia develops,* page 74.) The distinction between *acute* and *chronic* depends on rapidity of onset, disease progression, and cell maturity. Chronic leukemias *aren't* a chronic phase of acute leukemias. In *myelocytic* leukemia, granulocytes or monocytes proliferate. In *lymphocytic* leukemia, lymphocytes proliferate. Thus, the four major leukemia types are:
- acute myelocytic leukemia (AML)
- acute lymphocytic leukemia (ALL)
- chronic myelocytic leukemia (CML)
- chronic lymphocytic leukemia (CLL).

Subtypes within these categories reflect the precursor-cell stage at which leukemia arose. AML subtypes, for example, include acute

Continued on page 74

Leukocyte Disorders

How leukemia develops

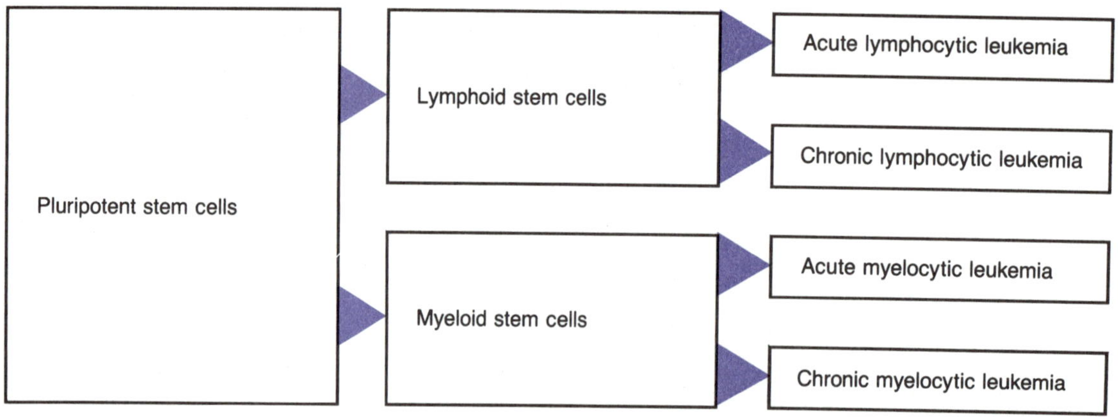

Leukemia—*continued*

myeloblastic leukemia, acute promyelocytic leukemia, acute myelomonocytic leukemia, acute monocytic leukemia, and erythroleukemia (a rare leukemia in which erythrocytes proliferate).

Leukemia classification by subtype proves useful because each subtype tends to affect a specific age-group, warrants a different drug therapy, and responds differently to treatment.

Acute leukemias have a rapid onset and progression. Immature, undifferentiated cells characterize these diseases. Untreated, acute leukemias typically lead to death within a few months. However, with treatment advances, many patients with acute leukemias survive longer than patients with chronic leukemias.

Chronic leukemias have a gradual onset and progression. In some patients, life expectancy may exceed 5 years. The relatively mature cells that predominate in chronic leukemias function more effectively than the more immature cells found in acute leukemias.

Acute leukemias are most common among children aged 2 to 4. The incidence declines by age 8, then rises again among persons age 65 and over. Chronic leukemias most frequently strike persons over age 20. Their incidence increases with age, peaking among those aged 60 to 70. Chronic lymphocytic leukemia rarely occurs in persons under age 45.

Assessment

Because anemia typically accompanies leukemia, stay alert for signs and symptoms of anemia when assessing your patient. Suggestive findings include fatigue, malaise, lethargy, edema, pallor, headache, tinnitus, dyspnea, palpitations, and, possibly, tachycardia and heart failure.

Your patient may report fever as the primary complaint—even if he doesn't have an obvious infection; the fever may be accompanied by night sweats. Check for mouth and throat ulcers; peritonsillar and perirectal abscesses; laryngitis; sinusitis; bronchitis; pneumonia; skin, nail, and urinary tract infections; and septicemia. Fungal infections, uncommon at leukemia's onset, increase in frequency as the disease progresses. Leukemia may also cause weight loss and heat intolerance (from increased metabolism).

Leukocyte Disorders

Common assessment findings in leukemia

Because leukemia can impair normal production of all blood cells, its signs and symptoms may reflect a deficiency of erythrocytes (causing anemia), leukocytes (causing infection), and thrombocytes (causing bleeding). Other clinical findings may arise from leukemic cell infiltration of bones and organs. Expect these signs and symptoms:

- abdominal fullness or pain
- abnormal masses
- bone or joint pain
- easy bruising or bleeding
- ecchymosis
- fatigue
- fever
- hepatomegaly
- infection
- lymphadenopathy
- petechiae
- purpura
- retinal hemorrhage
- splenomegaly
- sternal tenderness
- weight loss.

Decreased thrombocyte (platelet) production can result in abnormal bleeding. Ask your patient if he has frequent nosebleeds, experiences unusual bleeding after tooth extraction, or bruises easily. Ask a female patient about increased menstrual bleeding. Check for petechiae, oozing gums, retinal hemorrhage, and signs and symptoms of subarachnoid bleeding, for example, headache, visual disturbances, and unequal pupil size. (Intracranial, GI, or pulmonary bleeding can prove fatal.) As ordered, obtain stool and urine specimens to test for blood. (See *Common assessment findings in leukemia* for other signs and symptoms.)

Abdominal discomfort and bone pain may result from leukemic cell infiltration of the bone marrow, liver, spleen, and lymph nodes. Headaches, nausea, vomiting, diplopia, papilledema, cranial nerve palsies, and disorientation may signal increased intracranial pressure from meningeal infiltration. Decreased urine output may indicate renal insufficiency caused by kidney infiltration. Hyperuricemia (caused by either the disease or its treatment) can also lead to renal insufficiency. Some patients may report renal pain.

Diagnostic tests. To classify and stage the disease and establish the most effective treatment regimen, expect the doctor to order the following tests:

- *Complete blood count.* The patient's leukocyte count may be normal (5,000 to 10,000/μl), below normal (less than 1,000/μl), or extremely elevated (above 400,000/μl). Expect a below-normal platelet count and hemoglobin level. Abnormal leukocytes, including immature blast forms, may appear on a peripheral blood smear—myeloblasts with AML, lymphoblasts with ALL. An abnormal granulocyte predominance and the Philadelphia (PH^1) chromosome indicate CML; an abnormal lymphocyte predominance signals CLL.
- *Other blood tests.* Elevated blood urea nitrogen and creatinine levels may occur from renal insufficiency if leukemic cells have invaded the kidneys.
- *Lumbar puncture.* In about 5% of leukemia patients, lumbar puncture reveals abnormal leukocyte invasion into the CNS. This important finding may indicate the need for more aggressive therapy.
- *Radiographic tests and nuclear scans.* Chest and bone X-rays, nuclear scans, and computed tomography (CT) scans help detect leukemic lesions and infection sites. Gallium scans also can help identify such sites.
- *Lymphangiography and/or lymph node biopsy.* Although not performed routinely, these procedures can help locate cancerous lesions and accurately classify the disease. (For more information on these tests, see Chapter 2.)
- *Bone marrow aspiration and biopsy.* These procedures help confirm the diagnosis and identify the leukemic cell type. If aspiration doesn't yield an adequate marrow sample, the doctor may perform needle biopsy to obtain a bone fragment. Typical findings include marrow cell hyperplasia with an increased proportion of blood cell precursors. (For details on bone marrow aspiration and biopsy, see Chapter 2.)

Planning

The patient with leukemia presents challenging and complex nursing problems. Focus your interventions on promoting patient comfort;

Continued on page 76

Leukocyte Disorders

Leukemia—*continued*

minimizing adverse effects of chemotherapy; managing complications; preventing infection; maintaining fluid, electrolyte, and nutritional balance; performing good skin care; and providing psychological support and patient education. Because many leukemia patients are children, be especially sensitive to their emotional needs and those of their families.

Nursing diagnoses. Before determining your nursing care plan, develop the nursing diagnosis by identifying the patient's actual or potential problem, then relating it to its cause. Possible nursing diagnoses for a patient with leukemia include the following:
- infection (potential for); related to decreased leukocyte count and granulocytopenia
- activity intolerance; related to fatigue, malaise, and weakness secondary to leukemia and its treatment
- bowel elimination, alteration in (diarrhea); related to chemotherapy and/or radiation therapy
- skin integrity, impairment of (potential); related to chemotherapy and/or radiation therapy
- nutrition, alteration in (less than body requirements); related to the disease and its treatment
- fluid volume deficit (potential); related to vomiting and diarrhea secondary to chemotherapy and/or radiation therapy
- comfort, alteration in (pain); related to leukemic cell organ infiltration and invasive tests and treatments
- coping, ineffective family (compromised); related to leukemia, its treatment, and disruption of the family unit
- fear; related to life-threatening disease and its treatment
- self-concept (disturbance in body image); related to alopecia and the debilitating effects of leukemia and its treatment.

Sample nursing care plan: Leukemia

Nursing diagnosis	Expected outcomes
Nutrition, alteration in (less than body requirements); related to the disease and its treatment	The patient will: • state why he's losing weight. • explain ways to avoid excessive weight loss. • maintain adequate nutritional status.
Nursing interventions	**Discharge planning**
• Explain to patient the causes of his inadequate nutrition, such as nausea, vomiting, anxiety, anorexia, and mouth ulcers. • Evaluate the effectiveness of antiemetics and/or analgesics. • Provide a balanced diet with adequate protein, calories, vitamins, and minerals. • Offer small, frequent meals. • Let patient make his own food selections, within reason. • Serve food that's been prepared according to patient's tolerance for chewing, swallowing, and digestion. • Encourage fluids. • Monitor fluid intake and output and body weight. • Increase activity level as tolerated. • Give mouth care before and after meals. • Provide a calm environment during meals, undisturbed by tests and treatments whenever possible.	• Teach patient about basic food groups and identify foods high in protein, calories, vitamins, and minerals. • Provide written instructions explaining the action, administration schedule, dose, and adverse effects of any antiemetic and analgesic medications patient must take at home. • Teach patient how to recognize signs and symptoms of dehydration and advise him to contact the doctor if they occur. • Explain how physical activity relates to appetite. • Confer with dietitian to help patient and his family plan nutritious meals. • Consult community health nurse to check patient's nutritional status at home, as needed. • Refer patient and his family to a community organization, such as the American Cancer Society, for more nutritional information.

Leukocyte Disorders

The sample nursing care plan on the opposite page shows expected outcomes, nursing interventions, and discharge planning for one nursing diagnosis listed above the sample care plan. However, you'll want to tailor each care plan to fit your patient's needs.

Intervention

Treatment for acute leukemias aims to induce and maintain complete remission. The doctor will probably order chemotherapy (see *Chemotherapeutic agents used to treat leukemia*) and, in some cases, may perform bone marrow transplantation (see *Bone marrow transplantation,* page 79). A complication of bone marrow transplantation is graft-versus-host disease. (For more details see *Graft-versus-host disease,* page 80.)

With chronic leukemias, complete remission is so unusual that it's usually not attempted; chemotherapy rarely prolongs life. (However, bone marrow transplantation can improve survival odds for selected CML patients.) Therapeutic goals include normalizing the patient's leukocyte count and treating infection, bleeding, and other effects of the disease. See "Specific leukemia types" on page 78 for more information on treatment for the relevant type.

Nursing intervention. Because chemotherapy makes the patient extremely vulnerable to hemorrhage or infection, take the following measures when providing nursing care:
- Check the patient's vital signs every 4 hours.
- Assess him for signs of bleeding, for example, by observing his skin for petechiae and testing his urine and stool for occult blood.
- Take precautions to prevent bleeding, such as avoiding use of rectal thermometers and drugs and providing oral care with a soft toothbrush or swabs. Also avoid administering nonsteroidal anti-inflammatory drugs (NSAIDs), such as aspirin, and advise the patient to use an electric shaver instead of a razor.
- Follow the ordered schedule for administering antibiotics, to ensure proper blood levels.
- Monitor I.V. blood product administration, if indicated.
- Assess the I.V. chemotherapy site (if applicable) for signs of drug extravasation, such as redness, swelling, and tenderness. If extravasation occurs, stop the infusion, apply ice to the site, and infiltrate sodium bicarbonate or steroids subcutaneously, as ordered.

When teaching your patient about his disease, explain expected adverse reactions to chemotherapy, such as those arising from bone marrow suppression—for example, fever over 100° F. (37.8° C.), chills, swelling, sore throat, and cough.

Instruct the patient to watch for signs of thrombocytopenia (such as ecchymosis and petechiae), to immediately apply ice and pressure to any external bleeding site, and to avoid NSAIDs because they may cause bleeding. Also advise him to get adequate rest to counteract fatigue, and recommend a high-calorie, high-protein diet to minimize toxic chemotherapeutic effects.

Emphasize the importance of follow-up care and frequent blood tests, and advise the patient to take all medications exactly as prescribed. Teach him to recognize the signs and symptoms of disease recurrence (swollen lymph nodes in the neck, axillae, and groin and increased abdominal size or discomfort) and tell him to notify his doctor immediately if he detects these.

Continued on page 78

Chemotherapeutic agents used to treat leukemia

Alkylating agents
- busulfan (Myleran)
- chlorambucil (Leukeran)
- cyclophosphamide (Cytoxan, Neosar)
- uracil mustard

Antibiotic antineoplastic agents
- daunorubicin hydrochloride (Cerubidine)
- doxorubicin (Adriamycin)

Antimetabolites
- cytarabine [ARA-C, cytosine arabinoside] (Cytosar-U)
- mercaptopurine [6-MP] (Purinethol)
- methotrexate
- thioguanine [6-TG] (Lanvis)

Corticosteroids
- prednisone (Deltasone, Liquid Pred, Medicorten, Orasone, Prednicen-M, SK-Prednisone, Wojtab)

Vinca alkaloids
- vincristine sulfate (Oncovin)

Leukocyte Disorders

Leukemia—*continued*

Throughout your care, provide emotional support and be a good listener. Remember that the patient will probably be frightened and anxious. Remain flexible about visiting hours (especially with a child) to promote maximum interaction with his family and friends. With an elderly patient, try to keep his spirits up by improving his appearance, asking about his family, and providing a pleasant environment. For any patient, provide opportunities for favorite activities, if possible.

Prognosis. Various factors affect prognosis: the patient's age, clinical condition, leukemia type, and degree of leukemic cell infiltration into CNS structures and other body regions. Overall, the prognosis has improved steadily with advances in combination drug therapy and bone marrow transplantation.

Evaluation
Base your evaluation on the expected outcomes listed on your nursing care plan. To determine whether your patient has improved, ask yourself such questions as these:

- Can the patient explain how his weight loss relates to his disease?
- Does he know of ways to avoid excessive weight loss?
- Is his nutritional status adequate?

The answers to these questions will help you evaluate your patient's status and the effectiveness of his care. Keep in mind that these questions stem from the sample care plan on page 76. Your questions may differ.

Specific leukemia types

Acute myelocytic leukemia (AML)
AML involves the hematopoietic stem cell that differentiates into all myeloid cells (erythrocytes, granulocytes, monocytes, and thrombocytes). In this leukemia, myeloblasts—immature precursor cells—proliferate in the bone marrow, then invade the lymph nodes and spleen. Although AML occurs in all age-groups, it ranks as the most common leukemia in young adults.

Assessment. The patient with AML may have signs and symptoms of respiratory infection and anemia and may report bleeding from mucous membranes, sternal pain, headache, nausea, vomiting, or dizziness. The physical examination typically reveals hepatomegaly and splenomegaly.

Diagnostic tests. A WBC differential may show subnormal neutrophil and lymphocyte levels. Hematocrit and platelet levels typically drop below normal and Auer's bodies (thin, rodlike, cytoplasmic masses) appear microscopically. Bone marrow aspiration shows increased myeloblasts.

Intervention. Systemic chemotherapy aims to eradicate leukemic cells and induce remission by restoring normal bone marrow function. Chemotherapeutic agents used to combat AML include a combination of I.V. daunorubicin or doxorubicin, cytarabine, and oral thioguanine. If these fail to induce remission, the doctor may order a combination of cyclophosphamide, vincristine, prednisone, or methotrexate; high-dose cytarabine alone or with other drugs; amsacrine

Continued on page 81

Leukocyte Disorders

Bone marrow transplantation

In this procedure, bone marrow is aspirated from a donor, usually the patient's twin or sibling. The patient first receives chemotherapy, total body irradiation, or both, to kill any residual cancer cells. Then he's placed in protective isolation and receives the donated bone marrow by infusion, usually through a Hickman catheter. After 2 to 4 weeks, transplanted marrow should become engrafted. Until the new marrow functions, he receives transfusions of platelets, red blood cells, and possibly granulocytes to prevent hemorrhage and infection.

Candidates for the procedure include patients with diseases involving the marrow or other disorders for which aggressive therapy would cause marrow damage. These conditions include:
- leukemia (transplanted normal marrow replaces leukemic cells and marrow destroyed by intensive chemotherapy and/or irradiation)
- aplastic anemia (the transplant replaces diseased marrow that has lost its cell-generating capacity)
- immune deficiency diseases (the transplant replaces the patient's defective marrow).

Successful transplantation hinges on finding a compatible donor. Two major tests determine compatibility—the red cell antigen type (ABO and Rh) and the human leukocyte antigen (HLA) type (also called the white cell antigen test). The greater the compatibility, the greater the chance for success.

Donated bone marrow falls into these three categories:
- *autologous*—donated by the patient. Use of this marrow source eliminates the risk of graft-versus-host disease (GVHD), an immune response by donor marrow against the recipient. The newly generated cells enter the peripheral circulation and cause host-rejection symptoms, including maculopapular rash, pancytopenia, jaundice, joint pain, anasarca (generalized massive edema), and malnutrition.
- *syngeneic*—donated by an individual (almost always an identical twin) whose red cell and HLA antigens are identical to the patient's. Use of this marrow source also eliminates the risk of GVHD.
- *allogeneic HLA-match*—donated by an individual (usually a sibling) with the same HLA antigens as the patient. Use of this marrow source can lead to GVHD.

Complications. Besides GVHD, complications of bone marrow transplantation may stem from the high-dose chemotherapy and radiation that precedes marrow infusion. Infection is the major cause of death among transplant patients, but hemorrhage also poses a serious threat during the 4 to 6 weeks in which the patient experiences pancytopenia.

Nursing intervention. After the marrow infusion, take the following measures:
- Monitor the patient's vital signs every 15 minutes for 2 to 4 hours, then every 4 hours. Check for fever and chills, which may be the only signs of infection.
- Give prophylactic antibiotics, as ordered. To reduce the risk of bleeding, don't administer medications rectally or intramuscularly.
- As ordered, administer methotrexate, cyclosporine, or thalidomide (which is still experimental) to prevent GVHD. Watch for GVHD signs. If GVHD occurs, expect to administer corticosteroids and immunosuppressives, such as azathioprine, and I.V. fluids and hyperalimentation. Apply creams and ointments to relieve itching and discomfort.
- Administer vitamin and iron supplements, as ordered. Administer blood products, such as platelets and packed red cells, if ordered, based on daily blood test results.
- Give mouth care every 2 hours. Use hydrogen peroxide and nystatin mouthwash, for example, to prevent or treat candidiasis and other mouth infections. Also provide meticulous skin care, paying special attention to pressure points and open sites, such as aspiration and I.V. sites.

To obtain bone marrow from the donor, the doctor inserts a Jam-Shidi needle into the posterior iliac crest. The needle penetrates 1″ to 2″ (2.5 to 5 cm) through skin, fat, and muscle, then ¼″ (0.6 cm) into the bone.

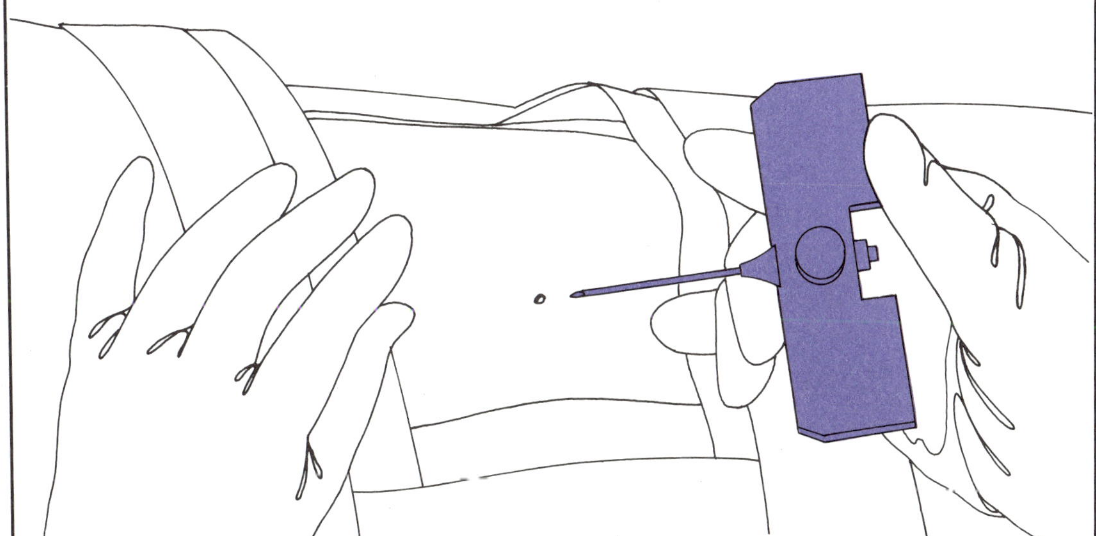

Leukocyte Disorders

Graft-versus-host disease

In graft-versus-host disease (GVHD), immunocompetent donor T lymphocytes attack and destroy vulnerable host cells. Because this disease occurs even with human leukocyte antigen (HLA) matching, non-HLA antigens may contribute to its development. Occurring most frequently in bone marrow transplants, GVHD affects the skin, liver, intestinal mucosa, and lymph system and may be acute or chronic.

Acute GVHD. Acute GVHD shows characteristic skin involvement and is confirmed by skin biopsy. Severe liver involvement also elevates liver enzyme and bilirubin levels.

Symptoms of acute GVHD occasionally appear as early as 1 week after transplantation, although 30 to 50 days is more typical. An erythematous rash appears first, followed by green, watery diarrhea, abdominal cramps, and, in severe disease, right upper quadrant pain, hepatosplenomegaly, jaundice, and enlarged lymph nodes.

Acute GVHD is graded according to the severity of symptoms and the number of organs involved. Patients with mild disease (Grade 1) experience skin involvement alone, whereas those with severe disease (Grades 2 to 4) also experience GI or liver involvement, which typically leads to fatal infection. Severe disease has an 85% mortality.

Treatment of acute GVHD includes high-dose corticosteroids, lymphocyte immune globulin, or cyclosporine. These agents may provide symptomatic relief, but their effectiveness in improving survival is still undetermined. In fact, corticosteroid therapy increases susceptibility to infection, the major cause of death in acute GVHD. Use of monoclonal antibodies to destroy donor T lymphocytes is still experimental.

Chronic GVHD. This form of GVHD may occur whether or not the patient experiences acute GVHD.

Chronic GVHD resembles autoimmune collagen vascular disorders, such as systemic lupus erythematosus. It's characterized by scleroderma-like skin fibrosis and Sjögren's syndrome, in which the mucosa and lacrimal ducts are abnormally dry. Diagnosis of chronic GVHD is confirmed by skin and oral mucosal biopsy. Also, Schirmer's test assesses lacrimal gland function and pulmonary studies measure pulmonary efficiency.

Chronic GVHD appears approximately 100 days after transplantation. It affects the skin, liver, GI system, oral mucosa, eyes, and vagina and causes pulmonary changes and muscle wasting.

Localized skin involvement may resolve without therapy. Treatment of early systemic involvement with combinations of immunosuppressive drugs shows promise but is still investigational.

Preventing GVHD. Immunosuppressive therapy against donor T lymphocytes aims to prevent GVHD. Methotrexate, an antimetabolite that inhibits DNA synthesis and has a cytotoxic effect on rapidly dividing cells, is the most commonly used therapy. Irradiation of blood products before they're administered also helps prevent T-lymphocyte replication.

Still experimental is the removal of T lymphocytes from the marrow before it's transplanted, by treating the marrow with monoclonal antibodies or by binding the T lymphocytes to plant substances called lectins.

Nursing intervention. Since patients with GVHD inevitably have some skin involvement, your major nursing goals are to maintain the integrity of the skin and mucous membranes and to prevent infection. Also strive to promote hydration and adequate nutrition to correct marked fluid and electrolyte losses caused by diarrhea and vomiting in severe disease. Monitor the patient with thrombocytopenia for GI blood loss.

Provide comfort measures to ease sore skin lesions, abdominal cramping, and pain. Also provide emotional support to the patient and his family.

GVHD stages according to organ system

Skin	Liver	Gastrointestinal
STAGE +1 Maculopapular eruption involving less than 25% of the body surface	STAGE +1 Moderate increase of serum glutamic-oxaloacetic transaminase (SGOT [150 to 170 IU]) and bilirubin (2 to 3 mg/dl)	Diarrhea, nausea, and vomiting are also Grades +1 through +4 in severity. Most of these manifestations, except diarrhea, are hard to quantitate.
STAGE +2 Maculopapular eruption involving 25% to 50% of the body surface	STAGE +2 Bilirubin rise (3 to 5.9 mg/dl) with or without an increase in SGOT	STAGE +1 500 ml of stool/day
STAGE +3 Generalized erythroderma	STAGE +3 Bilirubin rise (6 to 14.9 mg/dl) with or without an increase in SGOT	STAGE +2 1,000 ml of stool/day
STAGE +4 Generalized erythroderma with bulbous formation and, usually, desquamation	STAGE +4 Bilirubin rise (15 mg/dl) with or without an increase in SGOT (Increases in SGOT are temporarily related to the onset of worsening of the skin rash.)	STAGE +3 1,500 ml of stool/day STAGE +4 2,000 ml of stool/day

Grading GVHD

Grade 1 +1 to +2 skin rash with or without GI involvement
Grade 2 +1 to +3 skin rash with either +1 to +2 GI involvement or +1 to +2 liver involvement, or both; some patients have fever
Grade 3 +2 to +4 skin rash with +2 to +4 GI involvement with or without +2 to +4 liver involvement; many patients have fever
Grade 4 Similar to Grade 3 with extreme constitutional symptoms

Leukocyte Disorders

Specific leukemia types—*continued*

(experimental); or 5-azacytidine (experimental). Maintenance therapy involves additional chemotherapy.

Treatment may also include bone marrow transplantation and drugs to fight infection, such as antibiotics, antivirals, and antifungals. The doctor may order platelet transfusions to prevent bleeding and red blood cell transfusions to prevent anemia.

Prognosis. Untreated, AML commonly causes death within 2 to 3 months. Complete remission is the best predictor of a favorable outcome—patients who don't achieve complete remission after conventional chemotherapy have the same survival rate as those receiving no treatment. Although about 75% of AML patients achieve complete remission, relapses are common and subsequent remissions are usually brief. Overall, only about 20% of patients receiving conventional chemotherapy survive 5 years; about 50% of those patients who receive a bone marrow transplant from a matched sibling survive 5 years.

Several other factors help predict outcome. Although AML occurs more frequently in adults, children have a higher rate of complete remission. Longer remissions usually occur in patients showing Auer's bodies. Patients who develop AML after cytotoxic therapy for another disorder or after preleukemia (a period of leukemia-like symptoms of varying duration that precedes overt AML symptoms) have a poor prognosis.

Acute lymphocytic leukemia (ALL)
ALL results from a defect in a single lymphoid stem cell that produces clones that don't completely mature. These abnormal cells—varying from highly immature to almost normal—proliferate in the bone marrow, lymph nodes, and spleen. Prognosis varies according to the degree of cell maturity; a preponderance of highly immature cells predicts a poor outcome. The most common childhood leukemia, ALL accounts for about 10% of adult leukemia cases.

Assessment. The patient with ALL typically has a high fever of sudden onset. He may complain of headache, bone pain, and sternal tenderness. Thrombocytopenia causes abnormal bleeding (such as nosebleeds, gingival bleeding, or petechiae).

The physical examination typically reveals hepatomegaly, splenomegaly, lymphadenopathy, and ecchymosis. An internal eye examination may reveal retinal hemorrhages.

Diagnostic tests. Suggestive findings include subnormal neutrophil and hematocrit levels and platelet count and an elevated serum copper level. Also expect an increased overall leukocyte count. A blood smear typically shows immature lymphoblasts.

Intervention. The doctor will probably order systemic chemotherapy to eradicate leukemic cells and induce remission. Chemotherapeutic drugs used to treat ALL include vincristine and/or prednisone with intrathecal methotrexate or cytarabine; and I.V. asparaginase, daunorubicin, and doxorubicin. Treatment may also include antibiotic, antifungal, and antiviral drugs and granulocyte concentrate transfusions to control infection, platelet transfusions to prevent bleeding, and erythrocyte transfusions to prevent anemia. For maintenance

Continued on page 82

Leukocyte Disorders

Specific leukemia types—*continued*

therapy, expect the doctor to order mercaptopurine and methotrexate. In some cases, he may perform bone marrow transplantation.

Prognosis. Without therapy, an ALL patient typically dies within a few months—sometimes even a few days—from overwhelming infection or massive hemorrhage. However, intensive therapy improves the outlook, especially for children. A child who has remained in remission for 2 years after a 2½-year maintenance course has less than a 10% chance of relapse. This improved success rate results from advances in all treatment methods—chemotherapy, maintenance therapy, CNS prophylaxis, and supportive therapy for complications—since antileukemic therapy was introduced in 1948.

Achieving a complete remission is the key factor suggesting a good outcome; about 90% of children and 65% of adults achieve complete remission. Overall, the survival rate for ALL averages 18 months for adults and 36 to 42 months for children.

However, many patients, especially adults, suffer relapses. Cancerous cells may reappear in the bone marrow, CNS, or testes, even after maintenance therapy, CNS prophylaxis, and testicular irradiation. (CNS and testicular relapses have a rising incidence because more patients now survive longer.) Although subsequent remissions can occur, fewer patients achieve them and they're usually shorter than first remissions.

Besides complete remission, other factors—most importantly, age—affect outcome. Children between ages 3 and 7 have the best prognosis. Females have a better prognosis than males. Factors suggesting a poor outcome include obesity and CNS involvement, bleeding, or infection at diagnosis. Blacks and other nonwhites also have a worse prognosis. A high leukocyte count (above 100,000/μl) suggests a poor outcome because it may lead to cerebrovascular occlusion or hemorrhage.

Bone marrow transplantation during a second or subsequent remission increases life expectancy. About one third of children in second remission who receive transplants from a matched sibling remain alive 4 years later. By contrast, most children in second remission who *don't* receive transplants die within 3½ years.

Chronic myelocytic leukemia (CML)
CML involves the abnormal overgrowth of granulocytic precursors (myeloblasts, promyelocytes, metamyelocytes, and myelocytes) in bone marrow, peripheral blood, and body tissues. Rare in children, CML occurs most frequently in young and middle-aged adults. It affects slightly more men than women. In the United States, approximately 3,000 to 4,000 CML cases develop annually, accounting for roughly 20% of all leukemias.

CML's clinical course proceeds in two phases: the insidious *chronic phase,* with anemia and bleeding abnormalities and, eventually, the *acute phase (blast crisis),* in which myeloblasts—the most primitive granulocyte precursors—proliferate rapidly.

Almost 90% of patients with CML have the PH^1 chromosome. Discovered in 1960, this abnormality involves translocation of the long arm of chromosome 22, usually to chromosome 9. Radiation and carcinogenic chemicals may cause the condition.

Leukocyte Disorders

Blast crisis

Blast crisis eventually causes death in more than 70% of patients with chronic myelocytic leukemia (CML). In this disease phase, increasing numbers of blasts (immature myeloid precursor cells—especially myeloblasts, the most primitive granulocyte precursors) proliferate in the blood and bone marrow. Usually, blasts and promyelocytes (another myeloid cell precursor type) exceed 20% in the blood and 30% in the marrow. Increased fibrotic tissue in the marrow also suggests blast crisis. Leukopenia, thrombocytopenia, and anemia also appear.

Death usually occurs within 6 months after onset of blast crisis. However, bone marrow transplantation has improved the survival rate. Drug therapy that combines plicamycin and hydroxyurea may also extend the life of some patients. These drugs may destroy leukemic blast cells, transform them into normal granulocytes, or prevent the leukemic cells from inhibiting formation of normal granulocytes. Researchers are also investigating whether more aggressive therapies administered during CML's chronic stage can prevent progression to blast crisis.

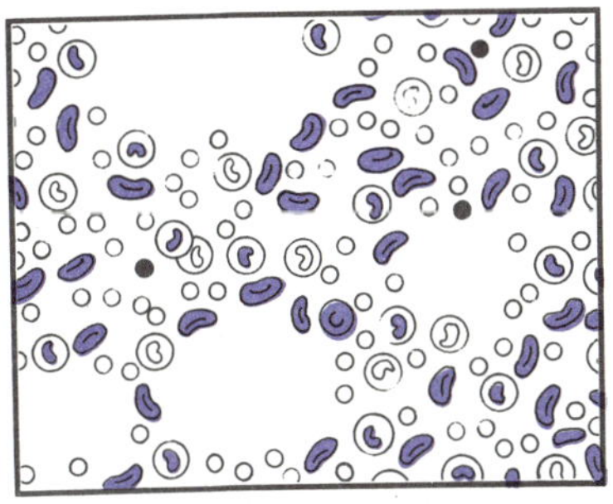

This microscopic view of a normal bone marrow specimen shows a normal distribution of blood cell types and fatty spaces. Note that blast cells appear in black.

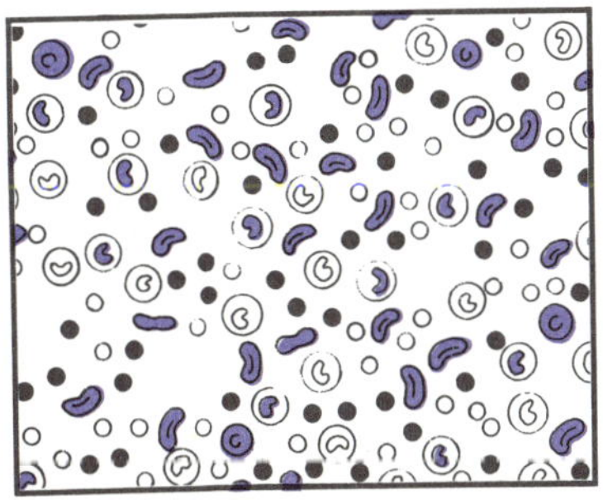

During blast crisis, the number of blast cells increases and fatty spaces shrink.

With blast crisis, CML takes on AML characteristics, with massive proliferation of promyelocytes and blasts in the bone marrow and blood. Anemia, fever, lymph node enlargement, splenomegaly, thrombocytopenia, thrombocytosis, or a suddenly elevated leukocyte count may signal the start of blast crisis. Random and unpredictable, blast crisis occurs annually in about 25% of patients diagnosed for more than 2 years.

Assessment. CML typically causes anemia signs and symptoms, including fatigue, weakness, pallor, headache, and dyspnea. Thrombocytopenia results in bleeding and clotting disorders, indicated by nosebleeds, gingival bleeding, hematuria, melena, ecchymoses, and easy bruising. The patient may also complain of severe abdominal discomfort and pain caused by splenic infarction from leukemic cell infiltration.

Other assessment findings may include sternal and rib tenderness from periosteal infiltration by leukemic cells; low-grade fever; weight loss; anorexia; renal calculi or gouty arthritis from increased uric acid excretion; and, occasionally, prolonged infection and ankle edema.

Diagnostic tests. In a patient with suggestive clinical findings, the PH_1 chromosome in peripheral blood or bone marrow and a low leukocyte alkaline phosphatase level confirm CML. Other relevant laboratory results include:

- leukocyte abnormalities—leukocytosis (leukocyte level above 50,000/µl, ranging up to 250,000/µl); occasional leukopenia (leukocyte level below 5,000/µl); neutropenia (neutrophil level below 1,500/µl) despite a high leukocyte count; and increased circulating myeloblasts
- hemoglobin level below 10 g/dl
- hematocrit value below 30%
- platelet count below 50,000/µl (however, the platelet count may be normal or even elevated)
- serum uric acid level possibly above 8 mg/dl
- bone marrow aspirate or biopsy revealing hypercellularity, with bone marrow infiltration by an increasing number of myeloid elements (biopsy is performed only if the aspirate's dry); in the acute phase, myeloblasts predominate.

Intervention. During CML's chronic phase, expect the doctor to order outpatient chemotherapy, usually including busulfan and, occasionally, melphalan, other nitrogen mustards, thioguanine, and hydroxyurea. Such therapy typically induces excellent remissions. Maintenance therapy may include low-dose outpatient chemotherapy.

Ancillary measures may include:

- local splenic radiation to reduce peripheral blood counts and spleen size, or splenectomy (controversial)
- leukapheresis (selective leukocyte removal) to reduce the leukocyte count
- bone marrow transplantation
- allopurinol to prevent hyperuricemia, or colchicine to relieve gouty attacks caused by an elevated serum uric acid level
- prompt treatment for infections that may result from chemotherapy-induced bone marrow suppression.

Continued on page 84

Leukocyte Disorders

Specific leukemia types—*continued*

During CML's acute phase, treatment resembles the regimen used for AML (although it's less likely to induce remission). It emphasizes supportive measures and chemotherapy with doxorubicin or daunorubicin, thioguanine, cyclophosphamide, vincristine, methotrexate, cytarabine, or daunorubicin with prednisone.

Prognosis. CML invariably proves fatal. Life expectancy averages 3 to 4 years after the chronic phase begins and 3 to 6 months after the acute phase starts. However, for patients who have matched siblings available as bone marrow donors, the outcome may improve considerably. Patients receiving transplants during the chronic phase have about a 40% to 50% 2-year survival rate; those receiving transplants during blast crisis have a 15% to 20% 2-year survival rate.

Age also affects life expectancy, with younger patients typically surviving longer. Other factors that tend to improve the prognosis include lack of the PH_1 chromosome, a leukocyte count below 100,000/µl, and normal liver function. On the other hand, patients with extremely high or low platelet counts have a poor prognosis, as do those with asthenia, bone pain, fever, GI problems, night sweats, and weight loss at diagnosis.

Chronic lymphocytic leukemia (CLL)
Characterized by the uncontrolled spread of abnormal, small lymphocytes in lymphoid tissue, blood, and bone marrow, CLL is the most benign and least progressive leukemia.

CLL accounts for almost one third of new leukemia cases annually. Life expectancy after diagnosis averages 3 to 6 years, although some patients live up to 20 years. Almost one third die from unrelated causes. Nearly all CLL patients are men over age 50.

Although CLL's cause remains unknown, researchers suspect still-undefined chromosomal abnormalities, hereditary factors (because of its higher incidence within certain families), and some immunologic defects, such as ataxia-telangiectasia or acquired agammaglobulinemia. CLL apparently *doesn't* result from radiation exposure.

Assessment. Signs and symptoms of CLL result from leukemic cell infiltration in bone marrow, lymphoid tissue, and organ systems. In early stages, the patient usually complains of fatigue, malaise, fever, and lymph node enlargement. He's particularly susceptible to infection.

In advanced stages, he may experience severe fatigue and weight loss, with liver or spleen enlargement, bone tenderness, and edema from lymph node obstruction. Pulmonary infiltrates may appear with lung parenchymal involvement. Skin infiltrations, manifested by macular to nodular eruptions, occur in about half of CLL patients.

As the disease progresses, bone marrow involvement may lead to anemia (indicated by pallor, weakness, dyspnea, tachycardia, and palpitations), bleeding, and infection. Opportunistic fungal, viral, and bacterial infections commonly occur in late stages.

Diagnostic tests. Typically, CLL's an incidental finding during a routine blood test that reveals numerous abnormal lymphocytes. In

Leukocyte Disorders

early stages, the leukocyte count remains mildly elevated, then rises as the disease progresses. The granulocyte count remains below normal. Other blood studies show a hemoglobin level under 11 g/dl, hypogammaglobulinemia, and a depressed serum globulin level. Other common findings include neutropenia, lymphocytosis (lymphocyte level over 10,000/μl), and thrombocytopenia (platelet count under 150,000/μl). Bone marrow aspiration and biopsy results show lymphocyte invasion.

Intervention. Because CLL occurs late in life and generally has a mild clinical course, treatment usually focuses on relieving symptoms and complications. However, in some cases, the doctor may order systemic chemotherapy involving alkylating agents—usually chlorambucil or cyclophosphamide—and sometimes steroids (prednisone), when autoimmune hemolytic anemia or thrombocytopenia occurs. If CLL causes obstruction or organ impairment or enlargement, local radiation can reduce organ size. The doctor may order allopurinol to prevent hyperuricemia, a relatively rare finding.

Prognosis. Death usually results from infection. Disease severity and response to therapy help predict outcome. Suspect a poor prognosis if your patient has anemia, thrombocytopenia, neutropenia, bulky lymphadenopathy, and severe lymphocytosis. Other factors indicating disease severity include the degree of fatigue, infections, masses, organ enlargement, and sternal tenderness.

Self-Test

1. To provide comfort for an anemic patient, appropriate nursing measures include all of the following except:
a. encourage the patient to alternate activity periods with rest **b.** turn him frequently to prevent skin breakdown **c.** clean his teeth with a firm toothbrush before and after meals **d.** serve frequent meals of soft, bland foods

2. Children who inherit the sickle-cell trait from one parent will usually develop the disease. True or false?
a. true **b.** false

3. Acute leukemias are most common in which one of the following age-groups?
a. ages 2 to 4 **b.** ages 10 to 20 **c.** ages 35 to 40 **d.** ages 50 to 60

4. Blast crisis occurs in which form of leukemia?
a. acute lymphocytic leukemia **b.** acute myelocytic leukemia **c.** chronic lymphocytic leukemia **d.** chronic myelocytic leukemia

Answers (page number shows where answer appears in text)
1. **c** (page 43) 2. **b** (page 57) 3. **a** (page 74) 4. **d** (page 83)

Congenital Coagulation Disorders: Hemophilia, Von Willebrand's Disease, and Other Problems

Brenda K. Shelton, who wrote this chapter, is a Research Nurse at the Veterans Administration Medical Center and University of Maryland Medical System, Baltimore. She received her BS from Towson State University, Baltimore. She has also earned her CCRN.

To maintain effective hemostasis—termination of bleeding by the body's coagulatory process—various vascular, platelet, and plasma factors must remain normal. Coagulation disorders can occur from an abnormality in any of these factors. Such disorders may result from congenital deficiencies or may arise as complications of other problems. In this chapter, we cover congenital coagulation disorders—hemophilia, von Willebrand's disease, and hereditary hemorrhagic telangiectasia. In Chapter 6, we discuss acquired coagulation disorders. (*Note:* Although thrombocytopenia is sometimes congenital, it's usually acquired; for this reason, we discuss it in Chapter 6.)

To increase your knowledge base and help you provide expert care for a patient with one of these problems, first review basics about platelets (thrombocytes) and the coagulatory process by reading what follows.

Platelet appearance and level. Platelets comprise the smallest formed blood element. Small, nonnucleated, and colorless, they usually appear as irregular spindles or ovals about 2 to 4 μm in diameter. They have a life span of 7 to 14 days.

Normal intravascular clot formation continuously consumes about 15% of circulating platelets. In adults, platelet counts normally range from 130,000 to 370,000/μl. Various factors influence this count. Epinephrine administration immediately raises it by about 30% to 50% (probably by mobilizing platelets from the spleen). Exercise can also increase the count. Because this happens even in a person who's had his spleen removed, experts believe that the lungs release some platelets into the circulation.

Normally, about 80% of platelets circulate through the bloodstream and about 20% remain in the spleen. Platelets move freely between the two sites; if the spleen enlarges markedly, up to 80% of the platelets may move into that organ.

Platelet functions. Platelets perform three vital functions:

- initiate contraction of damaged blood vessels to minimize blood loss
- form hemostatic plugs in injured blood vessels
- with plasma, provide materials that accelerate blood coagulation—notably platelet factor III.

Thrombopoiesis. Platelets descend from bone marrow precursor cells called megakaryocytes. Thrombopoietin, a humoral stimulating factor, regulates platelet production, which occurs mainly in the bone marrow (the lungs and spleen also produce some platelets).

Coagulation. When tissue or blood vessel injury occurs, changes in the body's vascular and extravascular tissue maintain hemostasis through a system of checks and balances. (See *Some conditions that trigger coagulation.*) The mechanisms involved include vasoconstriction, platelet plug formation, and blood clotting.

Vasoconstriction. Within seconds of vascular injury, neural reflexes and local smooth-muscle spasms cause the walls of the damaged vessel to contract. Constriction lasts about 10 minutes in a small

Congenital Coagulation Disorders

vessel and up to 30 minutes in a larger one. The extent of tissue damage determines the extent of vasospasm; for example, a blood vessel that suffers a clean cut bleeds more than one that is crushed. However, vasoconstriction slows blood flow only briefly in small vessels and can't prevent blood loss from large ones. Permanent repair requires a hemostatic plug formed of platelet aggregates and a fibrin clot.

Platelet plug formation. Normally, platelets circulate freely and don't adhere to one another or to the blood vessel's endothelial lining. But a blood vessel injury brings platelets into contact with the exposed collagen fibers and connective tissue beneath the endothelial lining. In response, platelets immediately change their features:

- They swell, taking on irregular shapes with numerous protruding processes.
- They become sticky, adhering to the collagen fibers.
- They secrete adenosine diphosphate (ADP), which, in turn, triggers swelling and adhesiveness in nearby platelets. These additional platelets then adhere to the originally activated ones. (Besides ADP, platelets release other chemicals during plug formation—for example, serotonin, which promotes vasoconstriction, and platelet factors III and IV, which promote coagulation.)

Thus, within seconds of injury, a platelet plug forms. With a minor injury, the plug may slow or stop bleeding completely. With more serious blood vessel damage, blood clotting may be necessary to restore hemostasis.

Blood clotting. This complex process involves various factors. First, it requires conversion of fibrinogen, a soluble protein normally present in the plasma, into fibrin, an insoluble, threadlike polymer. Fibrin threads form a meshwork that traps plasma, platelets, and other blood cells to form the clot. This conversion, in turn, requires activation of thrombin from prothrombin, an inactive plasma protein precursor.

Many reactions in the clotting process take place in a cascade—one component is triggered and, in turn, triggers another component, which then triggers yet another, and so on. In this rapid-fire fashion, inactivated factors in the blood become active clotting factors.

The cascade includes the intrinsic and extrinsic pathways, which merge into a common pathway. Vascular injury or foreign bodies in the circulation trigger the intrinsic coagulation system. Tissue injury stimulates the extrinsic coagulation system. The final common pathway begins as each pathway triggers the activation of factor X. For details in the sequence of events for normal clotting, from initial injury to clot formation, see *How a blood clot forms,* page 88, and *Understanding coagulation factors,* page 89.

Clot retraction and lysis (dissolution). Once activated, the various clotting factors are rapidly inactivated or removed by the blood to prevent widespread clotting. The clot then begins to retract. As its fibrin meshwork becomes stronger and denser, the injured vessel's edges pull closer together. Clot dissolution permits eventual clot breakdown. Within a few days after clot formation, plasmin acti-

Continued on page 89

Some conditions that trigger coagulation

Tissue injury
- burns
- surgery (especially cardiac and abdominal surgery)
- trauma (open or closed)
- necrotic processes (such as hepatitis and Crohn's disease)

Vascular injury
- surgery
- I.V. and intra-arterial line placement
- thrombotic damage to the vascular lining (such as from pulmonary emboli, myocardial infarction, or cerebrovascular accident)
- vascular malformation (such as from an aneurysm)

Foreign body within the vascular system
- emboli
- endotoxins from gram-negative organisms
- antigen introduction from anaphylaxis or transfusions of incompatible blood

Congenital Coagulation Disorders

How a blood clot forms

Vascular injury or foreign bodies in the vascular system or tissue injury initiate the blood-clotting mechanism. This involves a chain reaction of activated coagulation factors whose culmination is the formation of a blood clot.

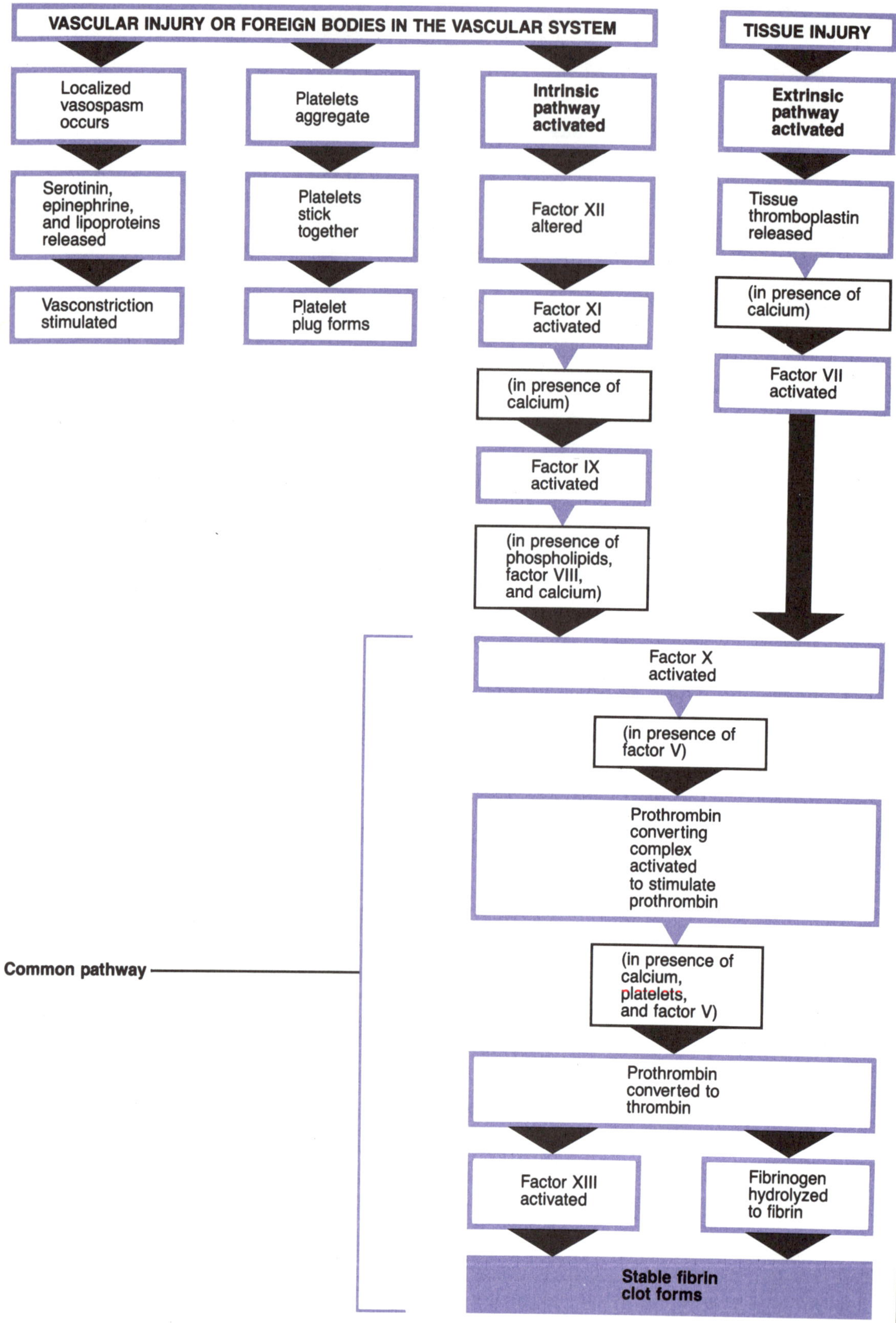

Congenital Coagulation Disorders

Continued

vators, which decompose fibrin, cause formation of enough plasminogen to dissolve the clot. By-products of clot dissolution are called fibrin degradation productions (FDPs, also known as fibrin split products [FSPs]).

Coagulation disorders. A deficiency or dysfunction in a specific portion of the clotting cascade characterizes various coagulation disorders. (See *Classifying coagulation disorders,* page 90.) Such disorders have varying clinical effects and necessitate different treatment. Most cascade-related disorders involve coagulation factor deficiencies or dysfunction. Congenital problems usually involve only one factor, whereas acquired disorders typically involve several. No matter which factor's deficient or dysfunctional, any interruption in the clotting cascade impairs hemostasis. (Certain anticoagulant medications act by blocking part of the cascade.)

Continued on page 90

Understanding coagulation factors

Factor	Synonym	Function	Synthesis site
I	Fibrinogen	Promotes normal platelet activity and wound healing	Liver
II	Prothrombin	Serves as inactive thrombin precursor	Liver
III	Tissue thromboplastin	Promotes prothrombin's conversion to thrombin in extrinsic clotting pathway	All tissues
IV	Calcium	Participates in or catalyzes several coagulation stages	From diet
V	Labile factor, proaccelerin	Accelerates prothrombin's conversion to thrombin in final common clotting pathway	Liver
VII	Proconvertin, stable factor	Promotes prothrombin's conversion to thrombin in presence of factor IV (extrinsic clotting pathway)	Liver
VIII	Antihemophilic factor	Promotes thromboplastin production and serves as procoagulant (participates only in intrinsic clotting pathway); deficiency results in hemophilia A (classic hemophilia)	Mononuclear phagocyte system
IX	Plasma thromboplastin component, Christmas factor	Influences thromboplastin amount (participates only in intrinsic clotting pathway); deficiency results in hemophilia B (Christmas disease)	Liver
X	Stuart-Prower factor	Permits intrinsic thromboplastin formation and prothrombin conversion; necessary in both intrinsic and extrinsic clotting pathways	Liver
XI	Plasma thromboplastin antecedent	Permits formation of prothrombin activator in intrinsic clotting pathway; deficiency causes hemophilia C	Unknown
XII	Hageman factor	Initiates intrinsic clotting pathway	Unknown
XIII	Fibrin stabilizing factor	Forms stabilizing bond within fibrin strands in final common clotting pathway	Unknown

Congenital Coagulation Disorders

Classifying coagulation disorders

Impaired coagulation component	Bleeding condition/disorder	Assessment findings
Vascular integrity	• Trauma to normal vessels • Vessel abnormalities caused by various diseases	• Pulsatile or flowing blood loss • Bright or dark red blood loss • Bleeding originating at or near recent vascular injury site or major vessel • Rapid symptom onset
Platelets	• Quantitative disorders (caused by platelet nonproduction, dilution, sequestration, or destruction) • Qualitative disorders (caused by abnormal platelet structure or drug intoxication, uremia, storage defects, or fibrin split products) • Combined quantitative and qualitative disorders	• Prolonged bleeding • Epistaxis or gingival bleeding • Easy bruising • Petechiae • Increased coagulation time after I.V. or intraarterial line insertion
Coagulation cascade	• Inactive factor disorders —congenital disorders (involving coagulation factors VIII, IX, and XI) —acquired disorders (such as impaired clotting factor production and vitamin K deficiency) • Active factor disorders —excessive heparin —excessive fibrin split products	• Prolonged bleeding • Bleeding disproportionate to extent of injury • Signs of occult blood in urine and feces • Easy bruising • Petechiae • Increase in bloody drainage • New bleeding from incision site
Clot lysis	• Abnormal fibrinolysis —administration of plasminogen activator (urokinase, streptokinase) —increased fibrinolysis secondary to increased fibrin formation	• Prolonged bleeding after injury • Severe tissue or vessel injury • Easy bruising • Petechiae

Continued

Cascade-related coagulation problems usually become noticeable only after blood vessel injury or tissue trauma. Laboratory studies can identify the specific coagulation defect.

Problems in the other components of the coagulation mechanism—blood vessels, platelets, and clot lysis—can also lead to coagulation problems. Most vascular coagulatory problems are caused by surgical or traumatic blood vessel damage, resulting in blood loss. The bleeding, which may be arterial or venous, varies in severity. Acute, severe vascular tears may cause rapid death; other tears may lead to prolonged obscure or minor symptoms.

The most life-threatening complication of bleeding from impaired vascular integrity is hypovolemic shock. For details on how to assess for and manage a patient with hypovolemic shock, see the NURSEREVIEW section on "Vascular Problems." Most platelet problems are characterized by small blood vessel bleeding in response to pressure, gravity, or minor trauma. Without normal platelet function, even minor capillary damage can cause blood leakage into interstitial tissues.

Platelet disorders fall into two groups: quantitative disorders (thrombocytopenias) involving abnormal platelet levels and qualitative disorders (thrombocytopathies) usually involving platelet dysfunction. Platelet disorders impair vascular integrity and the coagulation mechanism. However, serious coagulopathy is likely only when large numbers of platelets are dysfunctional or deficient.

Excessive or insufficient fibrinolysis (fibrin decomposition leading to clot removal) characterizes coagulation problems related to defective clot lysis. When a fibrin clot breaks down, FDPs continue

Congenital Coagulation Disorders

to circulate until the liver clears them. Normally, liver clearance takes place quickly. However, with severe liver disease or excessive FDPs, liver clearance decreases. Because FDPs are natural anticoagulants, abnormal bleeding or poor clot formation may result.

Laboratory FDP tests or ethanol gel tests can detect clot lysis syndromes involving excessive fibrinolysis. Disseminated intravascular coagulation (DIC) is the most common clot lysis disorder. (For information about DIC, read Chapter 6.)

Hemophilia

Hemophilia refers to a group of disorders characterized by coagulation factor deficiencies: hemophilia A (classic hemophilia—the most severe form) affects more than 80% of all hemophiliacs and results from factor VIII deficiency; hemophilia B (Christmas disease) affects about 15% of all hemophiliacs and results from factor IX deficiency; and hemophilia C, an even rarer form, results from factor XI deficiency. However, recent evidence suggests that hemophilia may result from *nonfunctioning* of factors VIII, IX, and XI, rather than from their deficiency.

All hemophilia forms are X chromosome–linked recessive disorders. Thus, a female carrier has a 50% chance of transmitting the defective X chromosome to each son; the affected sons will become hemophiliacs. She also has a 50% chance of transmitting the chromosome to each daughter; the affected daughters will become carriers. (See *Recognizing hemophilia inheritance patterns.*) A male

Continued on page 92

Recognizing hemophilia inheritance patterns

A sex-linked recessive disorder, hemophilia occurs almost exclusively in males; female carriers transmit the disease. As shown on the second line, each male offspring of a female carrier has a 50-50 chance of being born with hemophilia; each daughter has a 50-50 chance of being a carrier. The third line represents the third generation if the second generation offspring mate with normal partners.

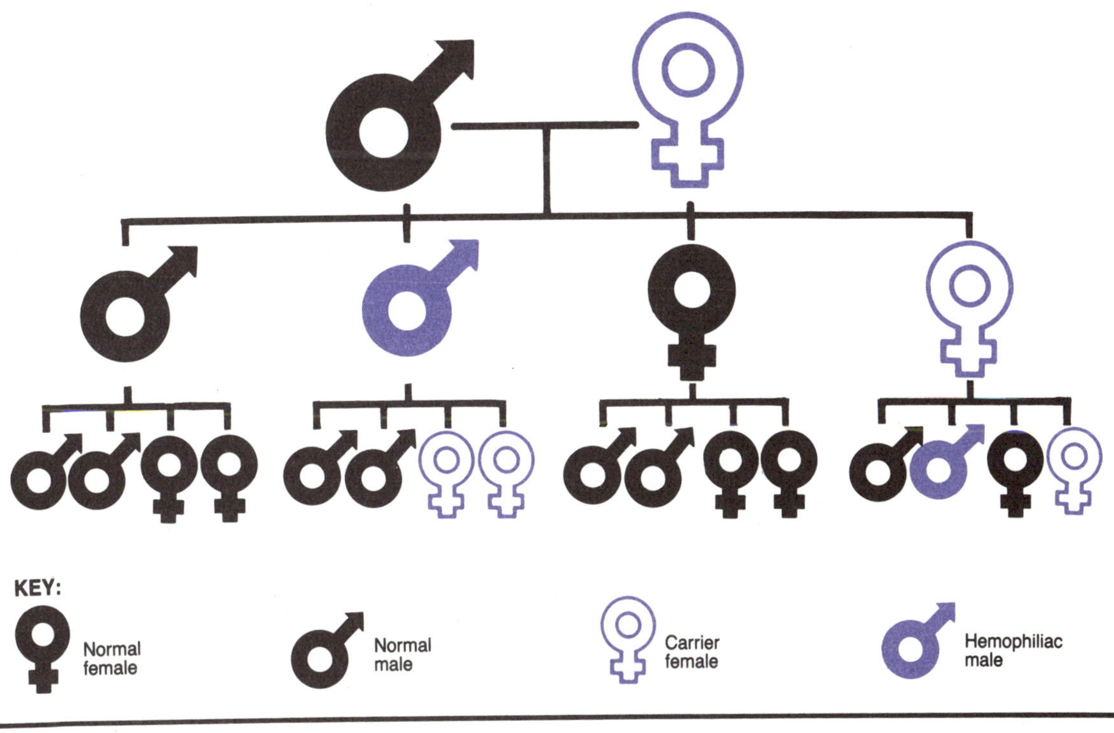

Congenital Coagulation Disorders

Hemophilia—*continued*

hemophiliac will transmit the X chromosome to his daughters, who will all become carriers. Female carriers rarely show any bleeding tendencies. However, as many as 30% of hemophiliacs have no notable family history; these cases may result from mutation in the genes that produce the involved coagulation factors.

In all hemophilia forms, patients have abnormal bleeding. Although a platelet plug forms at the bleeding site, the coagulation factor deficiency impairs the hemostatic response, preventing stable clot formation. Bleeding may be mild, moderate, or severe, depending on the degree of the factor deficiency (in VIII, IX, or XI) and on the bleeding site. (See *Factor VIII levels: Clues to bleeding severity.*)

Severe hemophilia may cause intracranial, GI, and renal hemorrhage. Hemarthrosis (blood extravasation into a joint or synovial cavity) can lead to joint pain and swelling in severe or moderate hemophilia (see *Hemarthrosis on X-ray*). Hemorrhage commonly occurs spontaneously or after minor or even imperceptible trauma. In descending order, the joints most commonly affected include knees, elbows, ankles, shoulders, hips, and wrists. An aura, indicated by tingling and warmth in the joint area, signals hemorrhage onset. This sensory symptom may last a few minutes to several hours, followed by joint movement limitation. Joint swelling and warmth may accompany severe joint movement limitation. Repeated episodes of hemarthrosis can destroy the joint, causing chronic disability.

Subcutaneous or muscular hematomas can result in pressure on vital organs, producing pain and functional limitations, as in hemophilia-induced renal failure. Hematomas may also impair peripheral nerve conduction, leading to peripheral neuropathies, paresthesias, and muscle atrophy.

Factor VIII levels: Clues to bleeding severity

Factor VIII level (% of normal)	Severity classification	Patient status
50% to 100%	Normal	No bleeding
25% to 50%	Normal to mild	May bleed excessively after major trauma
5% to 25%	Mild	May have severe bleeding after surgery or major trauma and some bleeding after minor trauma but doesn't bleed spontaneously
1% to 5%	Moderate	Severe bleeding after minor surgery and occasional spontaneous hemorrhages
Less than 1%	Severe	Frequent spontaneous bleeding into muscles and joints

Congenital Coagulation Disorders

Hemarthrosis on X-ray

As this illustration of an X-ray shows, hemophilia can cause soft-tissue swelling from hemorrhage into the joint space. Joint surface irregularities and cystic bone regions also appear.

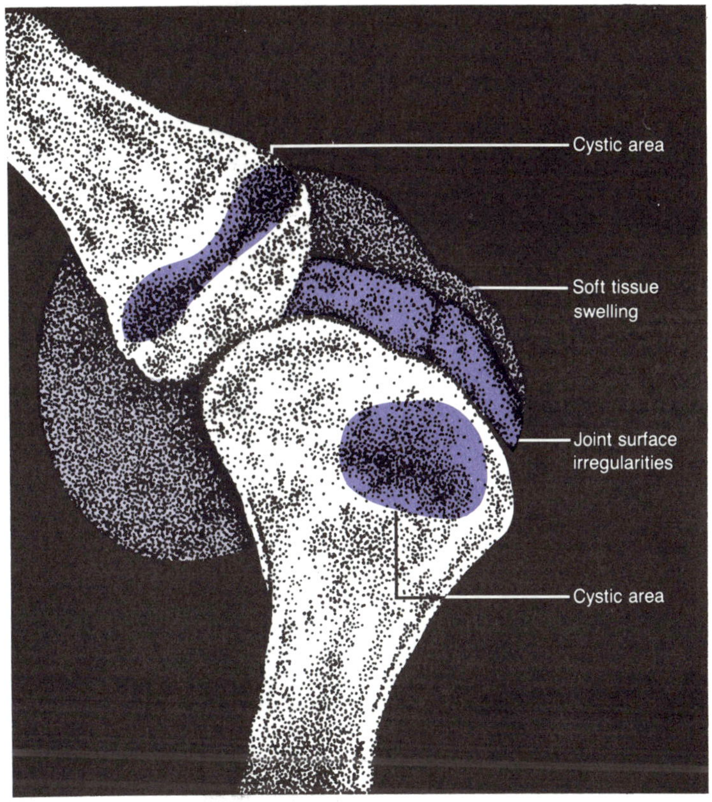

Assessment

Expect the hemophiliac patient to have a history of prolonged bleeding after trauma or surgery (including tooth extractions) or episodes of spontaneous bleeding into muscles or joints. However, mild hemophilia may remain undiagnosed until adulthood. Observe the patient with mild hemophilia for easy bruising, epistaxis, hematomas, and prolonged bleeding, especially after dental surgery. Postoperative bleeding typically continues as a slow ooze or stops and starts again, up to 8 days after surgery.

A positive family history can also help diagnose hemophilia. When taking the patient's history, determine if other family members have experienced bleeding problems or died of hemorrhage. If so, inquire about their age and their relationship to the patient and whether the bleeding problem was identified.

During an acute bleeding episode, expect some combination of the following:

- swollen painful joints
- local, persistent bleeding disproportionate to injury severity
- subcutaneous bleeding
- bleeding from mucous membranes
- abdominal pain and distention
- hematemesis or melena.

Continued on page 94

Congenital Coagulation Disorders

Hemophilia—*continued*

The first sign of severe hemophilia may be excessive bleeding after circumcision. Later, spontaneous or severe bleeding after minor trauma may produce large subcutaneous and deep intramuscular hematomas. Eventually, bleeding into joints and muscles can cause pain, swelling, and, possibly, permanent deformity.

Bleeding near peripheral nerves may lead to peripheral neuropathies, pain, paresthesias, and muscle atrophy. If bleeding impairs blood flow through a major vessel, it can result in ischemia and gangrene. Pharyngeal, lingual, intracardial, and intracranial bleeding may lead to shock and death.

Moderate hemophilia causes symptoms similar to severe hemophilia but produces only occasional spontaneous bleeding episodes.

Diagnostic tests. Characteristic laboratory findings in hemophilia A include:
- factor VIII assay 0% to 30% of normal
- prolonged activated partial thromboplastin time (APTT)
- normal platelet count, bleeding time (measures platelet function), and prothrombin time.

In hemophilia B, laboratory findings typically include:
- deficient factor IX assay
- baseline coagulation results similar to those found in hemophilia A, with a normal factor VIII level.

The degree of factor deficiency determines hemophilia's severity:
- mild hemophilia—factor levels more than 5% to 40% of normal
- moderate hemophilia—factor levels 1% to 5% of normal
- severe hemophilia—factor levels less than 1% of normal.

If bleeding complications exist, the doctor may order further tests, such as endoscopy for GI bleeding, computed tomography (CT) scanning to detect any intracranial bleeding, and arthroscopy or arthrography to identify certain joint problems.

Planning

Focus your nursing priorities on teaching the hemophiliac patient to avoid activities and conditions that can cause injury and bleeding—and subsequent illness and long-term complications. Also promote patient comfort and help him adjust his life-style to the limitations of his illness. Make sure he knows the signs and symptoms that warrant medical attention.

Nursing diagnoses. Before determining your nursing care plan, develop the nursing diagnosis by identifying the patient's actual or potential problem, then relating it to its cause. Possible nursing diagnoses for a patient with hemophilia include the following:
- injury, potential for; related to altered hemostasis
- tissue perfusion, alteration in; related to hemorrhage
- mobility, impaired physical; related to painful swollen joints
- comfort, alteration in (pain); related to hemarthroses
- activity intolerance; related to immobility
- anxiety; related to the risk of a bleeding episode
- fear; related to chronic disease and its treatment.
- coping, ineffective family (compromised); related to chronic illness

Congenital Coagulation Disorders

Sample nursing care plan: Hemophilia

Nursing diagnosis	**Expected outcomes**
Injury, potential for; related to altered hemostasis	The patient will: • identify activities or conditions that can precipitate bleeding. • compare symptoms of mild, moderate, and severe bleeding. • demonstrate local measures to stop bleeding. • describe bleeding characteristics that warrant medical management. • remain free from acute bleeding.
Nursing interventions	**Discharge planning**
• Monitor coagulation study results and blood product transfusions. • Inform patient and family about circumstances that can precipitate bleeding. • Teach them how to recognize bleeding signs and symptoms. • Teach them how to differentiate mild, moderate, and severe bleeding. • Instruct them when to seek medical help to control bleeding. • Advise patient to carry medical identification, to wear a Medic-Alert tag at all times, and to inform other health professionals, such as dentists, that he has hemophilia. • Develop a health maintenance regimen individualized to patient's needs.	• Provide written material to help teach patient and family about hemophilia and to reinforce teaching plan. • Answer any questions patient or family may have about treatment. • Review which medical treatments and procedures can trigger abnormal bleeding. • Evaluate knowledge and acceptance level of patient's support system. • Refer patient and family to a hemophiliac support group. • Provide patient and family with a source for obtaining factor VIII concentrate. • Arrange for consultation with a genetic counselor, as necessary.

• diversional activity, deficit; related to risk of bleeding
• knowledge deficit; related to genetic disease predisposition and medical treatment.

The sample nursing care plan shows expected outcomes, nursing interventions, and discharge planning for one nursing diagnosis listed above. However, you'll want to tailor each care plan to fit your patient's needs.

Intervention

Although hemophilia can't be cured, treatment can avert crippling deformities and lengthen life expectancy. The primary treatment—I.V. infusion of the deficient clotting factor—may be used to prevent bleeding after surgical or dental procedures or to stop bleeding from trauma.

For a patient with severe to moderate hemophilia A, the doctor may order infusion of factor VIII. Also called antihemophilic factor (AHF), factor VIII comes in two forms:
• single-donor, frozen concentrate, called cryoprecipitate (usually given by I.V. drip)
• commercially prepared freeze-dried concentrate extracted from large pools of plasma collected from paid donors. For more information on blood products and blood transfusions, see Chapter 3.

For a patient with mild hemophilia A, the doctor may order desmopressin instead of clotting factor concentrates. Desmopressin triggers release of stored factor VIII, temporarily doubling or tripling the patient's factor VIII level. As ordered, give the drug I.V. every other day for three or four doses.

For a patient with severe or moderate hemophilia B, the doctor usually orders freeze-dried prothrombin complex concentrate (which

Continued on page 96

Congenital Coagulation Disorders

Hemophilia—*continued*

includes factor IX) to prevent or treat bleeding. Given by I.V. push, this concentrate comes in a powder reconstituted with 20 to 30 ml of sterile water.

The doctor may treat a patient with mild hemophilia B with fresh-frozen plasma to lower the risk of exposure to hepatitis and other viruses. Each unit takes at least 30 minutes to infuse; an adult typically gets four or five units per infusion.

When a hemophiliac requires surgery, a hematologist with expertise in hemophilia should manage his care. The patient will require replacement of the deficient factor before and after surgery—sometimes even for such minor surgery as tooth extraction. To control oral bleeding, oral surgeons frequently use epsilon-aminocaproic acid, which inhibits the active fibrinolytic system.

Adverse effects of replacement therapy include allergic reactions to cryoprecipitate (for instance, pruritus, low-grade fever, urticaria, and bronchospasm). The major adverse effects of cryoprecipitate or factor VIII concentrate include exposure to hepatitis and human immunodeficiency virus (HIV), which causes acquired immune deficiency syndrome. Most treated hemophiliacs have plasma levels of hepatitis B surface antibody and the HIV antibody. However, the incidence of overt clinical hepatitis remains low. (*Note:* Most current preparation methods eliminate the risk of HIV transmission.)

Patients receiving large doses of factor IX concentrate have experienced deep vein thromboses and pulmonary emboli—especially with concomitant liver disease or after surgery and other conditions that increase the risk of thromboembolism.

Nursing intervention. During a bleeding episode, take these measures:

- Replace the deficient clotting factor or plasma, as ordered. The body metabolizes factor VIII in 4 to 24 hours, so repeat infusions, as necessary, until bleeding stops.
- Apply cold compresses or ice bags and elevate the injured area. (See *Agents for local bleeding management.*)
- To stop bleeding from recurring, restrict the patient's activities for 48 hours after bleeding has been controlled.
- Give such analgesics as acetaminophen, codeine, propoxyphene, or meperidine, as ordered, to control pain. *Don't* give I.M. injections, which may cause hematomas to form at the injection site. Avoid giving aspirin, ibuprofen, and compounds containing them; these drugs decrease platelet adherence and may promote bleeding.

If the patient has bled into a joint:

- Elevate the joint immediately.
- Initiate range-of-motion exercises, if ordered, at least 48 hours after bleeding has been controlled, to restore joint mobility. Instruct the patient to avoid weight bearing until the bleeding stops and swelling subsides.

Congenital Coagulation Disorders

Agents for local bleeding management

Most of these agents are applied locally to control surface bleeding and capillary oozing.

Agent	Possible indication	Application
Absorbable gelatin sponge (Gelfoam)	• Puncture wounds such as venipuncture, or bone marrow or tooth extractions	• Saturate foamlike wafers with isotonic saline injection or thrombin solution. • Apply pressure for 10 to 15 seconds. • Keep Gelfoam in place after bleeding is controlled.
Carafate (Note: Not an effective hemostatic but aids healing and promotes comfort)	• Oral and pharyngeal ulcers	• Crush sulfate tablets and mix with sterile water. • Instruct the patient to rinse his mouth or gargle with the solution.
Ice	• Large bleeding blood vessel • Hemarthrosis	• Apply ice pack to the site until bleeding subsides.
Microfibrillar collagen hemostat (Avitene)	• Surgery (hemostatic adjunct)	• Compress area with dry sponges. • Apply drug (amount depends on bleeding severity) with smooth, dry forceps to the bleeding site for 1 to 5 minutes. • Gently remove excess and reapply as needed.
Negatol (Negatan)	• Cervical bleeding (Note: Used more frequently with von Willebrand's disease)	• Insert 1-inch gauze packing dipped into 10% dilution of drug into cervical canal (may increase to full strength if tolerated). • Remove packing after 24 hours and give a 2,000-ml douche of dilute negatol or vinegar.
	• Oral ulcers	• Apply to dried oral lesions with an applicator. • Neutralize the negatol solution with large amounts of water.
Oxidized cellulose (Oxycel, Surgicel)	• Surgery (hemostatic adjunct) • External bleeding at tumor sites	• Apply with sterile technique (hemostatic effect is greater when applied dry). • Remove after hemostasis with dry sterile forceps (irrigate oxidized cellulose before removing to prevent fresh bleeding from occurring). • May leave in place if necessary.
Thrombin (Fibrindex, Thrombinar)	• Bleeding from: —parenchymal tissue —cancellous bone —dental, nasal, or laryngeal surgery —plastic surgery —skin-grafting procedures	• Apply 100 units/ml sterile isotonic saline solution or sterile distilled water to bleeding site (may apply powder to skin "brush burns"). • Apply 1000 to 2000 units/ml sterile isotonic saline solution to site for major bleeding. • Sponge blood from the site before application, but avoid sponging the area after the application (Note: May be used with absorbable gelatin sponge but not with oxidized cellulose [check sponge labeling before use]).
	• GI hemorrhage	• Give 60 ml (2 oz) of milk, followed by 60 ml of milk containing 10,000 to 20,000 units of thrombin. Repeat t.i.d. for 4 to 5 days or until bleeding is controlled.

After surgery or a bleeding episode:

- Carefully observe for signs of further hemorrhaging (for example, increased pain and swelling, fever, or evidence of shock).
- Closely monitor partial thromboplastin time (PTT).
- Teach the patient (or his family) specific precautions for avoiding bleeding episodes (see *Patient-teaching points,* page 98). Teach them

Continued on page 98

Congenital Coagulation Disorders

Hemophilia—*continued*

how to manage minor bleeding episodes and when to seek immediate medical attention. Reassure them that proper management will allow the child to lead a productive life.

• When caring for a child with newly diagnosed hemophilia, help him and his family adjust his life-style to his disease. The risk of bleeding excludes him from some early learning activities related to walking or climbing, restricting his ability to learn through play. Limiting his participation in such activities isolates him from other children. You can help him and his family acknowledge and cope with these problems by discussing them openly and, if necessary, referring them for counseling.

• Refer new or suspected hemophilia patients to a hemophilia treatment center for evaluation. Such centers can develop a treatment and management plan for the patient's primary-care doctor and serve as a resource for others involved in the patient's care, such as dentists or school personnel.

Evaluation

Base your evaluation on the expected outcomes listed on your nursing care plan. To determine whether your patient has improved, ask yourself such questions as these:

• Can the patient (or his family, if the patient's a child) name the activities that can precipitate bleeding?
• Can he distinguish between mild, moderate, and severe bleeding symptoms?
• Can he demonstrate how to stop bleeding by using local measures?
• Does he know when to seek medical help?
• Is he free from acute bleeding?

The answers to these questions will help you evaluate your patient's status and the effectiveness of his care. Keep in mind that these questions stem from the sample care plan on page 95. Your questions may differ.

Patient-teaching points

If you're caring for a patient with hemophilia, make sure you cover the following points when teaching him about his disease:

• Wear Medic-Alert jewelry and carry medical identification at all times.
• Avoid physical activities that increase the risk of blunt injury (such as most sports and heavy lifting and carrying).
• Maintain optimal physical and dental health.
• Avoid I.M. injections and inform any health professional who's drawing blood that you have hemophilia.
• Avoid using potentially harmful equipment (such as power tools and a safety razor).
• Avoid aspirin or ibuprofen products, which can cause bleeding.
• Wear gloves while gardening.
• Seek medical help to treat any bleeding that you can't manage at home.

Other congenital coagulation disorders

Von Willebrand's disease

An autosomal dominant or recessive inherited disease, von Willebrand's disease is characterized by prolonged bleeding time and factor VIII deficiency. Also known as angiohemophilia, pseudohemophilia, and vascular hemophilia, the disease affects more women than men. Although its incidence may exceed hemophilia's, it often remains undiagnosed until traumatic injury or surgery because it usually causes only mild symptoms. Experts believe that deficiency of a specific protein ($FVIII_{V}WF$) known to enhance both platelet adhesion and factor VIII activity causes von Willebrand's disease. Recently, scientists identified an acquired form of the disease in patients with cancer and immune disorders. An immunologic basis may underlie this acquired form, which causes rapid bleeding onset.

In most patients, bleeding results from a local cause, not a generalized clotting defect. In severe disease, bleeding episodes commonly begin early in childhood, then diminish with age. In moderate or mild cases, bleeding episodes may not appear until adulthood.

Congenital Coagulation Disorders

Von Willebrand's disease: Laboratory findings

- Prolonged bleeding time (more than 6 minutes)
- Slightly prolonged partial thromboplastin time (more than 45 seconds)
- Absent or reduced levels of factor VIII-related antigens (VIII_{AGN}), and low factor VIII activity level
- Defective in vitro platelet aggregation (using ristocetin coagulation factor assay test)
- Normal platelet count and clot retraction.

Assessment. Your patient may report bleeding or signs of bleeding (for example, epistaxis, gingival bleeding, bruising, and other mucosal and cutaneous bleeding). Menorrhagia's common in women with the disease and excessive postpartum bleeding occurs in about one of three affected mothers. GI bleeding commonly occurs—usually without an identifiable cause. Excessive bleeding may occur after surgery, such as tonsillectomy or tooth extraction. (Such bleeding sometimes leads to diagnosis of the disease.) Muscular hematoma and hemarthrosis are rare, helping to distinguish von Willebrand's disease from mild hemophilia.

Carefully assess the patient's previous response to trauma. If possible, find out if he bled from the umbilical cord after birth or from his penis after circumcision. Also ask about a family history of abnormal bleeding; typically, at least half the patient's family members share this tendency.

While performing the physical examination, check for spontaneous subcutaneous and mucous membrane hemorrhage, petechiae, and other superficial bleeding forms. Hemorrhage commonly begins seconds after injury and lasts for hours. Once it stops, however, it rarely recurs. If the patient's actively bleeding, carefully inspect all bleeding sites.

Diagnostic tests. Von Willebrand's disease may be difficult to diagnose because it usually causes mild symptoms and borderline laboratory values, including fluctuating factor VIII levels. However, in a patient with a positive family history and a characteristic bleeding pattern, laboratory studies can help establish the diagnosis. For typical laboratory findings, see *Von Willebrand's disease: Laboratory findings.*

Intervention. Local management—the preferred treatment for von Willebrand's disease—usually involves pressure, cold application, or a topical hemostatic agent. Should these measures fail, administer cryoprecipitate, as ordered, to ensure adequate levels of factor VIII polymer, which increases platelet adherence and decreases bleeding. Cryoprecipitate's effects last 4 hours; readminister the solution, as ordered, if bleeding continues. Some doctors also order a vasopressin (antidiuretic hormone) analog to enhance cellular release of stored factor VIII.

Nursing intervention. Make sure to provide nursing support during bleeding episodes, such as administering blood products, applying compresses, and monitoring laboratory values, as ordered. Also teach the patient how to maintain optimal health. Reassure him that bleeding episodes usually aren't severe or acute. If he must undergo invasive procedures or surgery, tell him that the doctor will probably order prophylaxis with cryoprecipitate to reduce the bleeding risk. Because the diagnosis of a bleeding disorder may make the patient fearful and anxious, help him set realistic activity restrictions. For example, remind him to take precautions against injury, such as by wearing shoes at all times, using a soft toothbrush, and shaving with an electric (not a safety) razor.

Hereditary hemorrhagic telangiectasia
Also known as Rendu-Osler-Weber disease, hereditary hemorrhagic telangiectasia (HHT) involves dilation of venules and capillaries.

Continued on page 100

Congenital Coagulation Disorders

Other congenital coagulation disorders—*continued*

This leads to formation of telangiectases, fragile masses of thin convoluted vessels that predispose the patient to hemorrhage. Hemangiomas—masses of blood vessels—may also appear. These localized, nonpulsatile, violet-colored masses bleed spontaneously. Frequently appearing flat or raised, they may blanch on pressure. (See *Identifying telangiectases and hemangiomas.*)

HHT affects both sexes but may cause less severe bleeding in females. Transmitted by autosomal dominant inheritance, it may be lethal in its homozygous state. Telangiectases may occur with such vascular malformations as arteriovenous fistulas. Visceral telangiectases commonly appear in the liver, bladder, respiratory tract, and stomach. Family members usually experience similar types of distributions of these lesions.

Generalized capillary fragility, manifested as spontaneous bleeding and spider hemangiomas of various sizes, may exist without overt HHT. Vascular malformation sometimes leads to pulmonary arteriovenous fistulas. In such cases, blood shunting through fistulas may cause hypoxemia, finger and toe clubbing, recurring cerebral embolism, and brain abscesses.

Assessment. Check your patient's face, ears, scalp, hands, feet, nasal and oral mucous membranes, and beneath his nails for characteristic telangiectases. Ask him if he has recently experienced epistaxis, hemoptysis, or GI bleeding (as indicated by hematemesis and melena). Because telangiectasia may lead to iron deficiency anemia, assess your patient for signs and symptoms of deficiency. In children, epistaxis is usually the first sign of HHT.

Identifying telangiectases and hemangiomas

Small red to violet lesions called telangiectases typically appear in patients with hereditary hemorrhagic telangiectasia (HHT). The lesions consist of thin, dilated vessels that may blanch on pressure and bleed spontaneously. They most commonly arise on the fingers, toes, lips, tongue, and oral and nasal mucous membranes.

A hemangioma, also called spider angioma, may also appear with HHT. This fiery red lesion, which reflects capillary fragility, has an elevated central body, branching spiderlike legs, and a surrounding flushed area. It may be singular or multiple and most commonly occurs on the face and neck (although rarely on the lips or ears).

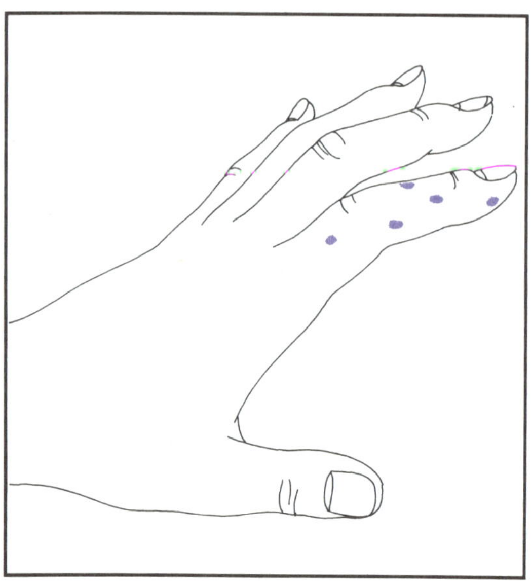

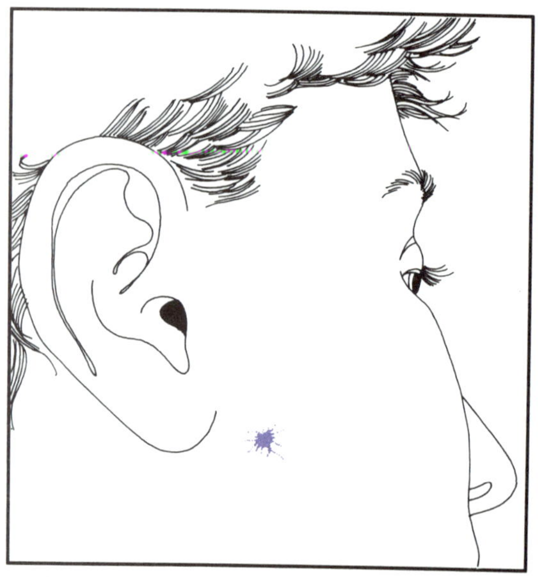

Congenital Coagulation Disorders

Diagnostic studies. Laboratory tests and bone marrow aspiration may reveal secondary iron deficiency anemia; red blood cells may be small and pale, indicating microcytic hypochromic anemia. Platelet function tests may be abnormal.

Intervention. Supportive therapy includes blood transfusions and parenteral iron supplements. Antipyretic or antihistamine administration before blood transfusion and use of saline-washed cells, frozen blood, or other preparations of leukocyte-poor blood may prevent febrile transfusion reactions. Parenteral iron enhances absorption to maintain sufficient iron reserves and prevents gastric irritation.

Nursing intervention. As ordered, apply topical hemostatic agents to bleeding sites and protect the patient from trauma and unnecessary bleeding. (The doctor may excise any accessible bleeding sites.) Also take the following measures:

- Observe the patient for signs of GI bleeding, such as hematemesis and melena. Advise him to watch for and report these signs.
- If the patient needs iron supplements, urge him to follow dosage instructions and to take them with meals to minimize gastric irritation. Warn him that iron turns stools dark green or black.
- Teach the patient and his family how to manage minor bleeding episodes—particularly recurrent epistaxis. Make sure they know when to seek emergency treatment.
- Refer the patient for genetic counseling, as appropriate.

Platelet function disorders

These disorders, which stem from platelet dysfunction, typically cause defects in platelet adhesion or procoagulation activity (ability to bind coagulation factors to their surface to form a stable fibrin clot). Such disorders may also create defects in platelet aggregation and thromboxane A_2 and may produce abnormalities by preventing the release of adenosine diphosphate (defective platelet release reaction).

Platelet function disorders may be congenital or acquired. Congenital disorders cause bone marrow production of platelets that don't clot effectively. Acquired disorders stem from the effects of drugs, such as aspirin or carbenicillin; from systemic diseases, such as uremia; or from other hematologic disorders.

Assessment. The first overt signs include sudden appearance of petechiae or purpura or excessive bruising and bleeding from the nose and gums. More serious effects are external hemorrhage, internal hemorrhage into the muscles and visceral organs, and excessive bleeding during surgery.

Diagnostic tests. These include prolonged bleeding time with both a normal platelet count and normal clotting factors. To determine the defective mechanism, the doctor will order a blood film and a platelet function test to measure platelet release reaction and aggregation. Depending on the type of platelet dysfunction, some or all test results may be abnormal. Other typical laboratory findings are poor clot retraction and decreased prothrombin conversion. Baseline testing includes complete blood count and differential and appropriate studies to determine hemorrhage sites.

Continued on page 102

Congenital Coagulation Disorders

Other congenital coagulation disorders—*continued*

Intervention. For congenital platelet dysfunction, platelet replacement is the only satisfactory treatment. Acquired disorders respond to adequate treatment of the underlying disease or discontinuation of damaging drug therapy. Plasmapheresis effectively controls bleeding caused by a plasma element that's inhibiting platelet function.

Nursing intervention. Keep these points in mind when caring for a patient with a platelet function disorder:

- Watch closely for bleeding from the skin, nose, gums, GI tract, or an injury site.
- Help the patient avoid unnecessary trauma. Advise him to tell his dentist about his condition before undergoing oral surgery.
- Alert other health team members to the patient's hemorrhagic potential, especially before he undergoes diagnostic tests that may cause trauma and bleeding.
- Observe the patient undergoing plasmapheresis for hypovolemia (indicated by hypotension and tachycardia), vasoconstriction, and other signs of volume depletion.
- If the platelet dysfunction is congenital, help the patient and family understand and accept the nature of this disorder. Teach them how to manage potential bleeding episodes. Warn them that petechiae, ecchymoses, and bleeding from the nose, gums, and GI tract should be reported immediately.
- Warn the patient to avoid aspirin, aspirin compounds, and other agents (such as ibuprofen) that impair coagulation.
- Advise the patient to wear a medical identification bracelet or to carry a card identifying him as a potential bleeder.

Acquired Coagulation Disorders: Thrombocytopenia, DIC, and Other Problems

Brenda K. Shelton, who wrote this chapter, is a Research Nurse at the Veterans Administration Medical Center and University of Maryland Medical System, Baltimore. She received her BS (nursing major) from Towson State University, Baltimore.

An acquired coagulation disorder can occur when a nonhereditary factor—for instance, medication, bone marrow suppression, excessive clotting factor consumption, or increased fibrinolysis—disrupts hemostasis. Usually complex, an acquired coagulation disorder may involve failure of any or all hemostatic components: vascular integrity, platelets, coagulation cascade, or clot lysis.

In this chapter, we'll cover the acquired coagulation disorders you'll encounter most frequently: immune thrombocytopenic purpura, disseminated intravascular coagulation, and coagulopathies related to vitamin K deficiency.

Immune thrombocytopenic purpura

The most common thrombocytopenia form, immune thrombocytopenic purpura (ITP) results from immunologic platelet destruction. A similar disorder, known as idiopathic thrombocytopenic purpura, is an autoimmune response similar to immune thrombocytopenia. Antibodies that reduce platelets' life span have been found in nearly all patients with either disorder. Although platelets retain their hemostatic role, they're destroyed by macrophages in the spleen because of their surface antigens.

ITP may be acute (known as postviral thrombocytopenia) or chronic (also called Werlhof's disease, purpura hemorrhagica, essential thrombocytopenia, and autoimmune thrombocytopenia). Acute ITP usually affects children between ages 2 and 9 (however, a disease identical to acute ITP can occur in adults); chronic ITP affects mainly adults under age 50, especially women between ages 20 and 40. ITP caused by drugs, allergies, or transfusions is generally chronic. Since sensitivity usually persists indefinitely, patients should avoid continued exposure.

Most common in the spring, acute ITP usually follows a viral infection, such as rubella, chicken pox, or a respiratory infection (a few patients have no clear history of viral infection). It can also arise after immunization with a live vaccine for chicken pox, mumps, measles, or smallpox. The link between infection and subsequent platelet destruction remains largely unknown, but scientists suspect that the infection causes an immune response that impairs platelets. Rarely, acute ITP follows blood transfusion, beginning about 1 week afterward and resolving spontaneously.

Most patients with acute ITP recover within 1 or 2 months. But a few develop acute hemorrhage, which may lead to fatal intracranial bleeding. This risk peaks during the first 2 weeks of the disease but may recur with severe thrombocytopenia.

Chronic ITP rarely follows infection. The doctor will probably diagnose this disorder if thrombocytopenia doesn't resolve after 6 months. Chronic ITP affects three times as many women as men and rarely occurs in blacks. Most common during young and middle adulthood, it can also strike the very young and very old.

Chronic ITP has recently been linked with other immune-related disorders, including sarcoidosis, Hodgkin's disease, non-Hodgkin's lymphoma, chronic lymphocytic leukemia, systemic lupus erythematosus, thyrotoxicosis, and possibly histoplasmosis, Hashimoto's

Continued on page 104

Thrombocytopenia: The most common bleeding disorder

Characterized by an abnormally low platelet count, thrombocytopenia can pose a serious threat to hemostasis. It can be congenital or acquired (more common) and results from decreased or defective platelet production in the bone marrow or increased platelet destruction. These abnormalities can develop secondary to various conditions, including:

- drug therapy, such as with gold salts, sulfonamides, antineoplastics, thiazide diuretics, or rifampin
- radiation therapy
- infection
- leukemia or aplastic anemia
- folic acid or vitamin B_{12} deficiency
- hypersplenism
- antibody-mediated platelet injury, which leads to immune thrombocytopenic purpura.

Bleeding severity depends on the patient's platelet count. With a count above 30,000/µl, he may bleed abnormally after surgery but won't bleed spontaneously. With a count between 15,000 and 30,000, expect mild spontaneous bleeding. With a count below 15,000, expect severe spontaneous bleeding. In drug-induced thrombocytopenia, the patient may recover immediately after the offending drug is withdrawn. Otherwise, the prognosis depends on the patient's response to treatment of the underlying cause.

Acquired Coagulation Disorders

Immune thrombocytopenic purpura: Recognizing possible causes

Food allergies
- Beans
- Citrus fruits

Diseases
- Certain cancers (including Hodgkin's disease, non-Hodgkin's lymphoma, and chronic lymphocytic leukemia)
- Hashimoto's thyroiditis
- Infectious diseases (such as chicken pox, mononucleosis, rubella, or viral hepatitis)
- Myasthenia gravis
- Sarcoidosis
- Scleroderma
- Systemic lupus erythematosus
- Thyrotoxicosis
- Tuberculosis

Medications
- Carbamazepine
- Digitoxin
- Gold salts
- Heparin
- Indomethacin
- Methyldopa
- Organic arsenicals
- Phenylbutazone
- Quinidine
- Quinine
- Rifampin
- Sulfonamides
- Thiazide diuretics

Toxic agents
- Insecticides
- Vinyl chloride

Transfusions (from antibodies to platelet antigen)

Vaccinations
- Chicken pox
- Measles
- Mumps
- Smallpox

Classifying your patient's hemorrhage risk

High risk
Platelets: 1,000 to 15,000/µl

Moderate risk
Platelets: 15,000 to 30,000/µl

Low risk:
Platelets: 30,000 to 100,000/µl

Drug-induced thrombocytopenia: Possible mechanisms

Some drugs may cause immune thrombocytopenic purpura by two proposed mechanisms. In the first (shown on the top), platelets become coated with the drug; the antibody then reacts with the platelet-drug complex. In the second proposed mechanism (shown on the bottom), the drug first combines with the antibody; then, the resulting drug-antibody complex coats the platelets.

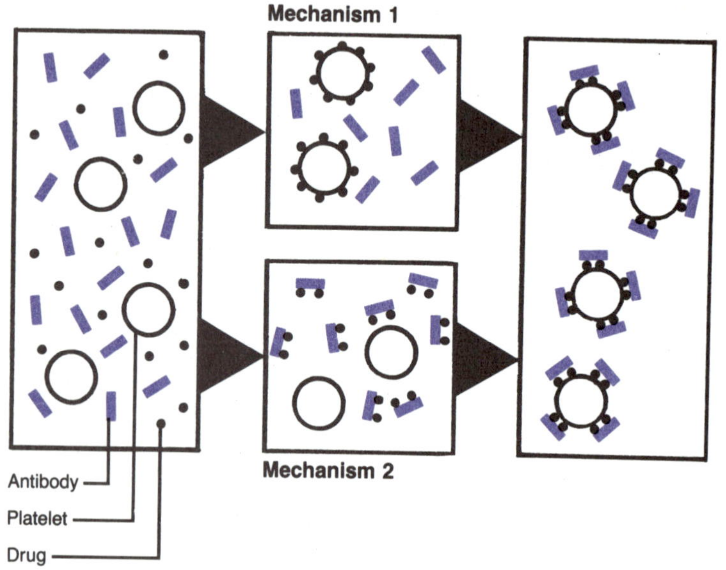

Immune thrombocytopenic purpura—*continued*

thyroiditis, scleroderma, myasthenia gravis, and some carcinomas. Experts don't know whether ITP precedes these diseases or results from their associated immune complexes.

Assessment

When taking your patient's history, ask about his health status, medication use, and exposure to toxic agents. Find out if he was recently immunized. Ask a female patient about excessive or prolonged menstrual bleeding. The patient may report general weakness, fatigue, malaise, and lethargy. Inquire about recent illness—acute ITP usually arises 2 to 21 days after a viral infection; however, in some cases, the interval between infection and the onset of purpura may be as long as 6 weeks.

Chronic ITP has an insidious onset. The patient may report evidence of minor bleeding—a bruising tendency or recurrent epistaxis—that began months or years before he sought medical help.

When performing the physical examination, check for petechiae and ecchymoses. Also stay alert for mucous membrane bleeding and hemorrhagic bullae (a sign of severe chronic ITP). Evaluate the patient for evidence of intracranial bleeding and increasing intracranial pressure—confusion, lethargy, and other level of consciousness changes; bradydysrhythmias; widening pulse pressure; projectile vomiting; and papilledema. You may detect liver and spleen enlargement and lymphadenopathy, probably reflecting recent viral infection in acute ITP.

Acquired Coagulation Disorders

Thrombocytopenia: Bone marrow findings

When thrombocytopenia results from accelerated platelet destruction, as in immune thrombocytopenic purpura, a bone marrow smear typically reveals increased numbers of megakaryocytes, as shown in this illustration. These giant platelet precursors may be less granular and have smoother contours than normal.

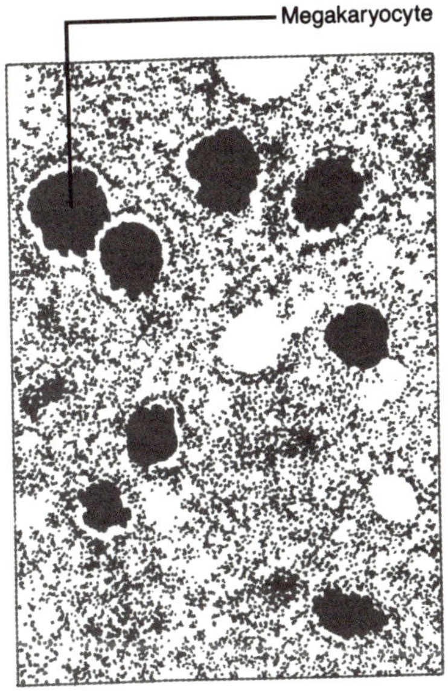

Identifying purpuric lesions

Petechiae are painless, round, pinpoint lesions, 1 to 3 mm in diameter. Caused by extravasation of red blood cells into cutaneous tissue (such as from thrombocytopenia), these red or brown lesions usually arise on dependent body regions. They appear and fade in crops and can group to form ecchymoses.

Ecchymoses, another form of blood extravasation lesions, are larger than petechiae. These purple, blue, or yellow-green bruises vary in size and shape and can arise anywhere on the body from trauma. Ecchymoses usually appear on the arms and legs of patients with thrombocytopenia or other bleeding disorders.

Diagnostic tests. With acute ITP, expect severe thrombocytopenia initially—a platelet count below 20,000/μl—and prolonged bleeding time. Platelets may be abnormal in size but have a normal morphologic appearance. Anemia may appear if the patient has lost blood. Bone marrow studies may show abundant megakaryocytes (platelet precursors). Other findings include decreased platelet survival time (several hours or days rather than the usual 7 to 10 days), decreased clot retraction, and increased capillary fragility. Platelet antibodies may be found.

With chronic ITP, the platelet count is subnormal but usually somewhat higher than with acute ITP (possibly up to 75,000/μl). Other laboratory findings resemble those found with acute ITP.

Planning

Focus your nursing care on reducing the bleeding risk, detecting early bleeding signs, and intervening appropriately. Also take measures to maintain optimal patient health.

Nursing diagnoses. Before determining your nursing care plan, develop the nursing diagnosis by identifying the patient's actual or potential problem, then relating it to its cause. Possible nursing diagnoses for a patient with acute or chronic ITP include the following:

- injury, potential for (bleeding); related to decreased platelet count and/or shortened platelet survival time
- comfort, alteration in (pain); related to hemorrhage
- thought processes, alteration in; related to intracranial bleeding
- tissue perfusion, alteration in (cerebral); related to intracranial bleeding
- oral mucous membrane, alteration in; related to injury and coagulopathy
- tissue integrity, impaired; related to bleeding
- knowledge deficit; related to effects of bleeding tendency and ways to prevent injuries that cause bleeding
- coping, ineffective individual (potential); related to bleeding tendency.

The sample nursing care plan on page 106 shows expected outcomes, nursing interventions, and discharge planning for one nursing diagnosis listed above. However, you'll want to tailor each care plan to fit your patient's needs.

Intervention

Acute ITP. To reduce bleeding severity, the doctor may order platelet transfusions, which may temporarily help a patient with severe hemorrhage. Although rapidly sensitized and removed by the liver, transfused platelets may promote hemostasis. Plasmapheresis (therapeutic plasma exchange) offers another treatment option for those severely affected. This procedure removes the patient's plasma (which contains immune complexes causing ITP) from the blood and replaces it with fresh normal plasma.

Gamma globulin administration, an experimental treatment, can help elevate the platelet count and reduce platelet turnover. Glucocorticoids, such as prednisone, have been used with mixed success; for a child, the doctor will probably order these drugs only after splenectomy.

Continued on page 106

Acquired Coagulation Disorders

Sample nursing care plan: Immune thrombocytopenic purpura

Nursing diagnosis	Expected outcomes
Oral mucous membrane, alteration in; related to injury and coagulopathy	The patient will: • describe signs and symptoms of oral bleeding. • be able to differentiate between mild, moderate, and severe bleeding. • state when he should seek medical help.
Nursing interventions	**Discharge planning**
• Teach patient to recognize signs and symptoms of bleeding and have him name those that require medical treatment. • Monitor complete blood count and coagulation studies for signs of blood loss and coagulopathy. • Check patient's mouth for lesions and bleeding after giving oral care. • Assess patient daily for petechiae, bruising, and oozing blood. • Instruct patient to use a soft toothbrush and to avoid flossing, if possible.	• Reinforce patient teaching and provide patient and family with written materials. • Remind patient to use a soft toothbrush and to avoid flossing. Review proper use of Stimudent. • Evaluate level of patient's and family's knowledge of bleeding signs and symptoms. • Advise patient to tell his dentist about his bleeding problem. • Arrange for appropriate follow-up health care and diagnostic tests.

Immune thrombocytopenic purpura—*continued*

Regardless of the treatment used, up to 90% of patients with acute ITP recover within 6 months. ITP that doesn't improve by then is considered chronic and may warrant splenectomy. (However, the doctor won't remove the spleen of a child under age 4.)

Chronic ITP. Expect the doctor to order glucocorticoids—usually prednisone—as the first therapeutic choice. As ordered, begin the drug at 0.5 mg/kg, increasing to 1 mg/kg as needed and to 2 mg/kg if platelet count is below 10,000/µl. Once the patient's platelet count has stabilized at about 50,000/µl, reduce the dose gradually, as ordered, over several weeks. If the patient needs excessive doses to maintain an acceptable platelet count, or if the count doesn't rise after 2 to 3 weeks of therapy, expect the doctor to perform a splenectomy. Alternatively, he may order an immunosuppressive drug such as azathioprine or cyclophosphamide given concomitantly with prednisone, or vincristine given alone. Because such drugs can cause infection and even cancer, the doctor will carefully weigh their potential benefits against these risks.

Other treatments that may be used in an attempt to manage chronic ITP include plasmapheresis and gamma globulin administration. About 10% to 20% of patients with chronic ITP recover without treatment.

Nursing intervention. Care for the ITP patient as you would for any patient who's bleeding or at risk for bleeding. To control bleeding, use specific measures, such as applying pressure or giving transfusions, according to bleeding severity. Also try to prevent injuries and other situations that could precipitate bleeding by taking the following measures:

- Restrict the patient's activities to avoid even minor trauma.
- Elevate the head of his bed.
- Maintain adequate oral prophylaxis to prevent gingivitis.
- Advise the patient to use a soft toothbrush.
- Give stool softeners, as ordered, to avoid constipation.

Acquired Coagulation Disorders

- Pad bed rails or place pillows under the patient's limbs.
- Avoid limb dangling for long periods.
- Administer saline nasal spray to reduce nasal irritation from dry air and to avoid nasal encrustation.
- If the patient's unsteady on his feet, help him perform activities of daily living.
- Use caution when administering sedatives, which can cause injury from impaired motor function.
- Avoid giving aspirin and other drugs that suppress platelet function.
- Avoid I.M. and subcutaneous injections.
- Draw blood only when necessary and avoid other invasive procedures whenever possible.
- Instruct the patient to avoid using straight razors.

Evaluation

Base your evaluation on the expected outcomes listed on your nursing care plan. To determine whether your patient has improved, ask yourself such questions as these:

- Can the patient identify signs and symptoms of bleeding?
- Can he tell the difference between mild and severe bleeding?
- Does he know when to obtain medical help for bleeding?

The answers to these questions will help you evaluate your patient's status and the effectiveness of his care. Keep in mind that these questions stem from the sample care plan on page 106. Your questions may differ.

Disseminated intravascular coagulation

Disseminated intravascular coagulation (DIC), also known as consumption coagulopathy, defibrination syndrome, and intravascular coagulation with fibrinolysis, is characterized by uncontrolled clotting in the microcirculation. Normally, bleeding causes changes that trigger the coagulation cascade, in which a system of checks and balances regulates clotting. In DIC, these regulatory mechanisms fail and clotting accelerates, resulting in clots in the capillary bed where they're not needed. This causes depletion of certain coagulation factors; because of this depletion, clots can't form where they *are* needed. Clot-dissolving mechanisms begin dissolving even stable clots before the body can replace the missing coagulation factors. As a result, anticoagulant factors become overabundant, triggering uncontrolled hemorrhaging. Thus, paradoxically, bleeding and clotting occur at the same time. Small vessels become occluded, possibly leading to tissue ischemia and organ necrosis. Because the process occurs throughout the circulation, all organs are vulnerable.

DIC always arises as a complication of other diseases and conditions. These primary disorders stem from three basic pathologic processes:

- tissue injury, which activates the coagulation cascade's extrinsic pathway and leads to release of thromboplastin and other procoagulants. This occurs, for example, with certain cancers and after surgery.
- vascular endothelial injury, which triggers the coagulation cascade's intrinsic pathway. Such injury can result from shock, amniotic fluid embolism, prolonged cardiopulmonary bypass surgery, adult respiratory distress syndrome, infection, and other conditions.

Continued on page 108

Thrombocytosis and thrombocythemia

Indicated by a platelet count above 800,000/μl, *thrombocytosis* is usually temporary and commonly follows severe hemorrhage or surgery (especially splenectomy). It may also accompany iron deficiency and some neoplastic disorders. A platelet count that persistently stays above 1 million/μl indicates *thrombocythemia,* which signals a myeloproliferative disorder (for example, chronic lymphocytic leukemia or polycythemia). The patient may have spontaneous bleeding secondary to leakage from damaged vessels, thrombosis, necrosis of vessels distal to clots, and splenomegaly. Anticoagulants are usually the drugs of choice for treatment.

Acquired Coagulation Disorders

How DIC develops

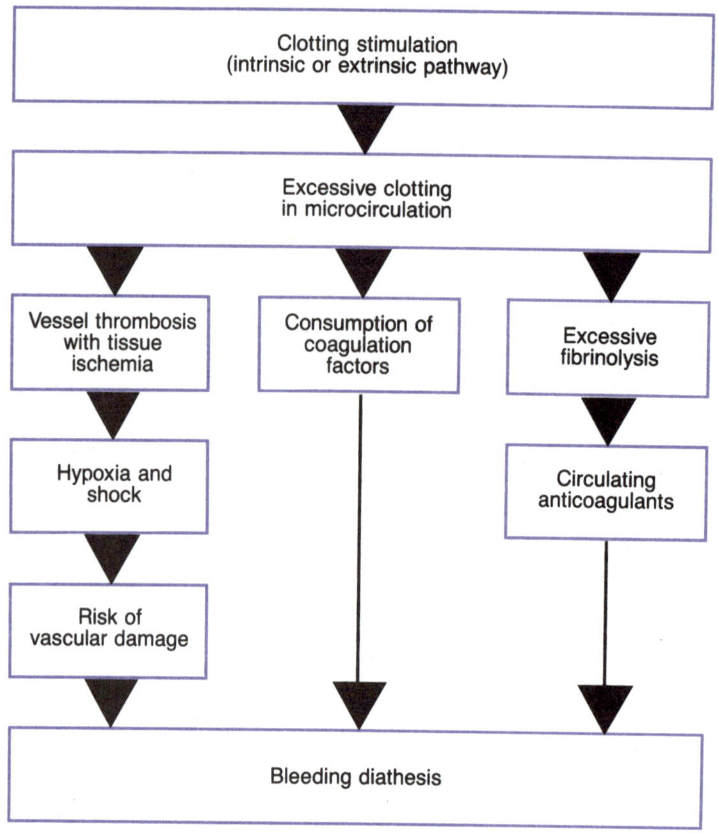

Disseminated intravascular coagulation—*continued*

• foreign body in the bloodstream, which triggers the coagulation cascade's intrinsic pathway. This injury may occur with transfusion reactions, gram-negative sepsis and endotoxins, pulmonary or venous emboli, and amniotic fluid embolism.

Although DIC commonly has a rapid onset, symptoms and generalized body involvement may not always seem acute. Chronic subclinical DIC may develop in patients with chronic procoagulant stimulation (also called a hypercoagulable state), as in chronic vascular disorders.

Assessment

Abnormal bleeding without an accompanying history of a serious bleeding disorder is the hallmark of DIC. Check for signs of such bleeding, including cutaneous oozing, petechiae, ecchymoses, hemorrhagic bullae, and wound hematomas. Also inspect for bleeding from surgical or invasive procedure sites and from the GI tract, as well as for signs of acute tubular necrosis.

To assess for signs of occult bleeding, examine the patient's abdomen for distention and test excreta (sputum, vomitus, urine, and stool) for occult blood. Note any skin color changes, malaise, weakness, altered sensorium, vision changes, headache, dyspnea, orthopnea, and tachycardia. Consider acrocyanosis—sharp, irregular demarcation of peripheral cyanosis—a key finding, indicating fibrin deposition in the microcirculation.

Acquired Coagulation Disorders

How DIC affects blood clots

In this illustration of an arteriole, overabundant anticoagulant factors destroy red blood cells and dissolve a stable clot.

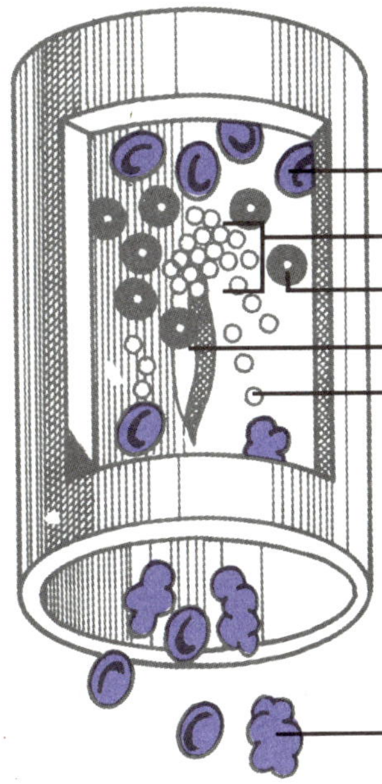

DIC: Identifying associated disorders

- Abruptio placentae
- Adrenal disease
- Adult respiratory distress syndrome
- Amniotic fluid embolism
- Anaphylaxis
- Anoxia
- Burn injury
- Diabetic ketoacidosis
- Drug reactions
- Eclampsia
- Fat embolism
- Graft-versus-host disease
- Head trauma
- Heat stroke
- Hypoxia
- Infection (particularly with gram-negative organisms)
- Kidney disease
- Liver disease
- Major surgery
- Massive trauma
- Neoplastic disease (especially leukemias, lymphomas, and solid lung, breast, and prostate tumors)
- Placenta previa
- Prolonged cardiopulmonary bypass surgery
- Pulmonary embolism
- Retained fetal tissue and placenta
- Shock
- Sickle-cell anemia
- Snakebite
- Transfusion reactions

To assess for impaired tissue perfusion, check for decreased blood pressure; confusion; restlessness; syncope; abnormal behavior; dyspnea; tachypnea; and decreased urine output. Other possible effects of DIC include nausea; vomiting; severe muscle, back and abdominal pain; convulsions; coma; shock; and major organ failure. Stay especially alert for these problems in a patient who's at risk for hypotension, capillary blood stasis, hypoxemia, or acidosis. (For a complete list of signs and symptoms, see *DIC assessment findings,* page 110.)

Diagnostic tests. Laboratory tests, while valuable, may show few abnormalities until DIC has progressed to end-organ involvement. Diagnosis may be hard to confirm because similar findings occur in other disorders. Initial results supporting a tentative DIC diagnosis include:

- platelet count below 100,000/μl
- fibrinogen level below 195 mg/dl
- prothrombin time (PT) longer than 15 seconds
- partial thromboplastin time (PTT) longer than 60 seconds
- fibrin degradation products (FDPs) greater than 45 mcg/ml (possibly above 100 mcg/ml).

Other supportive data include positive fibrin monomers, diminished Factor V and VIII levels, fragmented red blood cells, and a decreased hemoglobin level (below 10 g/dl). Renal function tests may show an elevated blood urea nitrogen level (above 25 mg/dl) and an elevated serum creatinine level (above 1.3 mg/dl). Urinary output may drop below 30 ml/hour. To help identify the underlying disorder, the doctor may order further tests. Final confirmation of the diagnosis may be difficult, since many of these tests are used to diagnose other diseases.

Continued on page 111

Acquired Coagulation Disorders

DIC assessment findings

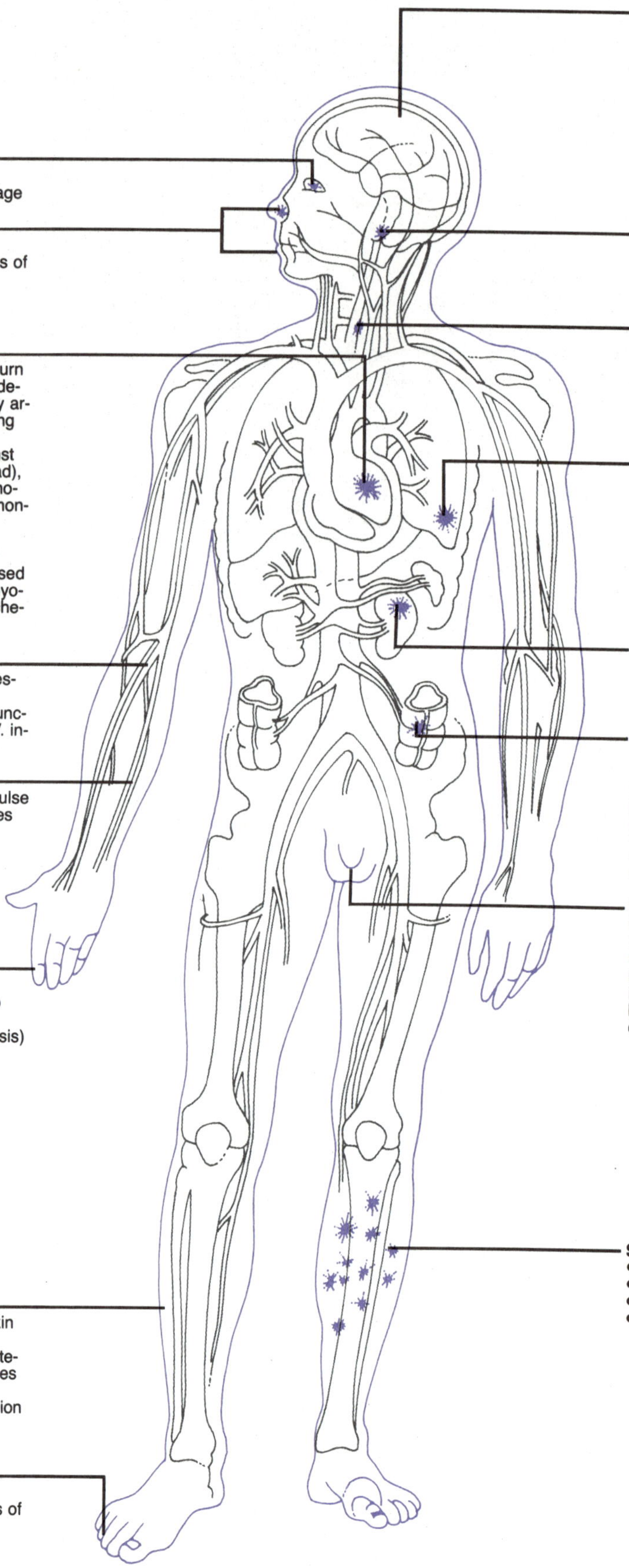

Acquired Coagulation Disorders

Disseminated intravascular coagulation—*continued*

Planning

Focus your nursing care on identifying early signs and symptoms of DIC and the underlying disorder, correcting anemia and hypovolemia, and preventing further bleeding.

Nursing diagnoses. Before determining your nursing care plan, develop the nursing diagnosis by identifying the patient's actual or potential problem, then relating it to its cause. Possible nursing diagnoses for a patient with DIC include the following:

- breathing pattern, ineffective; related to tachypnea
- cardiac output, alteration in (decreased); related to reduced central venous, pulmonary artery, and pulmonary capillary wedge pressures
- tissue perfusion, alteration in; related to hypovolemia
- fluid volume deficit (actual); related to uncontrolled bleeding
- injury, potential for (trauma); related to clotting problem
- urinary elimination, alteration in patterns; related to progressive oliguria
- comfort, alteration in (pain); related to blood engorgement
- communication, impaired (verbal); related to aphasia
- fear; related to rapid disease onset
- thought processes, alteration in; related to intracerebral bleeding.

The sample nursing care plan below shows expected outcomes, nursing interventions, and discharge planning for one nursing diagnosis listed above. However, you'll want to tailor each care plan to fit your patient's needs.

Continued on page 112

Sample nursing care plan: Disseminated intravascular coagulation

Nursing diagnosis	**Expected outcomes**
Tissue perfusion, alteration in; related to hypovolemia	The patient will: • maintain adequate heart rate and rhythm, blood pressure, and central venous pressure. • maintain fluid balance. • show signs of improved circulation. • display signs of improved respiratory status.
Nursing interventions	**Discharge planning**
• Monitor heart rate and rhythm, central venous pressure, blood pressure, and respiratory rate and depth every hour until patient's stable, then every 2 to 4 hours. Record and report any changes. • Measure and record urinary output every hour until it exceeds 30 ml/hour, then progress to every 2 to 4 hours. • Monitor patient for signs and symptoms of fluid imbalance and transfusion reaction. • Initiate measures to help improve perfusion, such as keeping patient warm and relieving pain and anxiety. • Perform chest physiotherapy with caution and encourage patient to cough and deep-breathe.	• Refer patient to psychiatric nurse practitioner, social worker, or other resource person to provide emotional support at home. • Consult with community health nurse to ensure continued health care. • Review care plan and teaching plan with patient and family. Answer questions. • Teach patient how to use pressure, cold compresses, and topical hemostatic agents to control bleeding at home. • Advise patient when to seek medical help to control bleeding. • Arrange for follow-up medical appointments.

Acquired Coagulation Disorders

Disseminated intravascular coagulation—*continued*

Intervention

Expect the doctor to order measures aimed at correcting the underlying disorder. Provide general supportive care, as ordered, including administering replacement fluids and ensuring adequate oxygenation and blood pressure. Further treatment depends on the patient's response. For example, you may administer heparin to reverse life-threatening or progressive microvascular occlusions. Heparin interferes with the coagulation cascade at several stages, antagonizing thrombin production and preventing clot formation and secondary activation of the fibrinolytic system. (*Note:* Although heparin inhibits clot formation, it has no effect on formed clots.) The drug also inhibits further microcirculatory fibrin deposition and prevents platelet agglutination. Thus, it promotes fibrinolysis while improving brain, kidney, and skin perfusion. However, heparin therapy is controversial because it impedes clotting and, consequently, may exacerbate bleeding. If this occurs, you may need to administer platelets and plasma clotting factors, which DIC depletes. Heparin also can cause anaphylaxis and may induce delayed thrombocytopenia (after 9 to 12 days of therapy). Rarely, it may induce antiplatelet antibody production and thrombus formation.

As ordered, regulate the heparin dose to double the total clotting time or to increase the PTT to 2½ times normal. Follow a bolus I.V. injection of 10,000 units or more with intermittent I.V. injections or continuous I.V. administration. The patient may require unusually high heparin doses to correct intravascular clotting.

If your patient has life-threatening or excessive bleeding that hasn't responded to treatment, the doctor may order a fibrinolytic inhibitor (such as aminocaproic acid [Amicar]) to block accumulation of circulating FDPs. However, these drugs can also cause inappropriate clot lysis (concomitant heparin administration may help counteract this effect).

Nursing intervention. Use standard measures to control bleeding. Monitor the patient's laboratory values, especially platelet count, fibrinogen level, PT, plasma thrombin time, and FDPs, to evaluate therapeutic effectiveness. If the doctor orders blood products, administer them according to hospital policy and procedure. As ordered, initiate measures to reverse multisystemic failure. For details on nursing intervention, see *Managing DIC.*

Evaluation

Base your evaluation on the expected outcomes listed on your nursing care plan. To determine whether your patient has improved, ask yourself such questions as these:

- Does the patient have adequate heart rate and rhythm, central venous pressure, and blood pressure?
- Can he maintain fluid balance?
- Has his circulation improved?
- Has his respiratory status improved?

The answers to these questions will help you evaluate your patient's status and the effectiveness of his care. Keep in mind that these questions stem from the sample care plan on page 111. Your questions may differ.

Managing DIC

Follow these guidelines when caring for a patient with DIC:

- Carefully check blood study results, especially hemoglobin and hematocrit values and coagulation times.
- Give replacement blood or blood products, as ordered. Watch for transfusion reactions and fluid overload.
- Assist with mechanical ventilation, peritoneal dialysis, or hemodialysis, as ordered.
- Administer oxygen, as ordered.
- Determine your patient's blood loss by weighing the dressings and linen; record the amount of drainage. *Note:* Don't forget to include blood specimens when you document blood loss.
- Weigh the patient at the same time each day and in the same or similar clothing to check his fluid balance —particularly if he has a kidney disorder. In acute DIC, monitor intake and output hourly.
- Watch for bleeding from the gastrointestinal and genitourinary tracts. If you suspect intraabdominal hemorrhage, measure the patient's abdominal girth every 4 hours. Test specimens of gastric secretions, stool, and urine for blood.
- Stay alert for signs and symptoms of hypovolemic shock.
- Check I.V. sites frequently for bleeding.
- Limit I.M. and subcutaneous injections. Apply pressure to injection sites for at least 10 minutes to control bleeding.
- To prevent blood clots from dislodging and causing fresh bleeding, don't scrub bleeding areas.
- Use pressure, cold compresses, and topical hemostatic agents, such as an absorbable gelatin sponge (Gelfoam), to control bleeding.
- If ordered, give your patient heparin and/or aminocaproic acid (Amicar). *Note:* Heparin's contraindicated if the patient has brain damage or dysfunction or if he has a necrotizing lesion.
- Protect your patient from injury. Turn and position him carefully. Enforce bed rest during bleeding episodes and pad the bed's side rails if your patient's agitated.
- Provide gentle mouth care. Remember, your patient's gums may bleed easily.
- Avoid using adhesive tape. The force needed to remove it may damage skin, causing bleeding.
- To help control pain from tissue ischemia, administer analgesics

continued

Acquired Coagulation Disorders

Managing DIC—*continued*

that do not contain aspirin, as ordered.
- Perform passive range-of-motion exercises on your patient during nonbleeding periods to reduce joint and muscle pain. Avoid giving back rubs or skin massages because these may promote bleeding.
- Because DIC may cause hemorrhaging in major organs, watch your patient for signs and symptoms of cerebral, gastrointestinal, and hepatic hemorrhage.
- Provide emotional support for the patient and his family.

Coagulopathies related to vitamin K deficiency

Vitamin K is essential to liver synthesis of prothrombin and coagulation factors VII, IX, and X (commonly called the vitamin K–dependent coagulation factors). Consequently, a vitamin K deficiency can cause abnormal bleeding. Because various foods and the intestinal flora contain vitamin K, primary deficiency from insufficient dietary intake occurs only in unusual circumstances—for example, in a severely malnourished patient who's receiving antibiotics. A disorder resembling vitamin K deficiency develops among newborns in the first few days of life, from liver immaturity, poor placental vitamin K transfer, or inadequate intestinal vitamin K production.

In adults, vitamin K deficiency usually arises secondary to disease or drug therapy, for instance:
- decreased bile flow to the small intestine, from a bile duct obstruction or biliary fistula
- malabsorption syndromes, including cystic fibrosis, sprue, and pellagra
- bowel resection, ileitis, or ulcerative colitis
- chronic liver disease with impaired liver enzyme response to vitamin K
- prolonged use of anticoagulants that counteract vitamin K, or broad-spectrum antibiotics (including penicillins and cephalosporins), which destroy the intestinal flora. Read on to review details on two of these causes.

Liver disease. Because the liver synthesizes clotting factors, vitamin K–dependent chronic liver disease can lead to vitamin K deficiency by impairing such synthesis. Other hemostatic abnormalities associated with liver disease include:
- reduced plasma levels of factors II, V, VII, and X
- development of coagulatory inhibitors
- excessive fibrinolysis.

Anorexia, poor food selection, and malabsorption can exacerbate vitamin K deficiency secondary to liver disease. Because most of these patients have concomitant gastritis, esophageal varices, or peptic ulcer disease, GI bleeding commonly signals a coagulation problem.

Anticoagulant therapy. Oral anticogulants (such as dicumarol and warfarin) suppress liver synthesis of certain clotting factors. Vitamin K antagonists, these drugs help manage thromboembolic disease, including pulmonary embolism and deep vein thrombosis, and may be ordered after coronary artery bypass surgery, valve replacement, aortic aneurysm repair, and other grafts or prosthesis implantation.

Up to 25% of patients receiving oral anticoagulants develop bleeding problems. In a patient on well-controlled anticoagulant therapy, the problem usually appears after trauma or development of a local lesion (for example, a duodenal ulcer). Bleeding without vascular injury most commonly stems from an increased anticoagulant effect caused by excessive anticoagulant administration or drug interaction.

Continued on page 114

Acquired Coagulation Disorders

Vitamin K deficiency: Common assessment findings

- Patient either young or elderly
- Concomitant drug therapy—antibiotics, antiplatelet agents, heparin, or oral anticoagulants
- Gastrointestinal disease
- Liver disease
- Malabsorption syndromes
- Kidney disease
- Surgery

Coagulopathies related to vitamin K deficiency—*continued*

Assessment

When taking your patient's history, look for clues to a possible vitamin K deficiency. Inquire about his past and present health and nutritional status, recent surgery, and medication use. Stay alert for complaints of prolonged bleeding after minor injury, easy bruising, mucosal bleeding, epistaxis, hematemesis, hematuria, or melena.

During the physical examination, check for petechiae, ecchymoses, and oozing blood. Palpate the patient's liver and spleen and note any enlargement; inspect his stools for overt blood or test them for occult blood. In a newborn, check for bleeding from the umbilical cord and also for intracranial bleeding.

Laboratory findings that suggest vitamin K deficiency include a prolonged PT (possibly an early sign that precedes bleeding) and, in severe deficiency, a prolonged PTT. In a patient with liver disease, also expect these other laboratory abnormalities:

- increased fibrinolysis, indicated by an elevated FDP level
- decreased platelet count
- subnormal fibrinogen level (with advanced liver disease).

Common anticoagulants and fibrinolytics: Monitoring therapy

If your patient's receiving anticoagulant or fibrinolytic therapy, monitor his coagulation test values and check for signs of drug toxicity, as shown by abnormal bleeding. Notify the doctor at once if you discover a problem. He may order the appropriate antidote listed below.

Drug	Test to determine toxicity	Antidote
dicumarol (Dicumarol Pulvules)	PT	• Phytonadione (vitamin K_1 [AquaMEPHYTON, Konakion, Mephyton]) • Menadiol sodium diphosphate (vitamin K_3 [Synkayvite])
heparin (Heparin Lock Flush Solution [Tubex], Hep-Lock, Liquaemin Sodium)	PTT	• Protamine
Recombinant tissue plasminogen activator/rTPA (Activase)	PT, PTT	• Fresh whole blood or fresh frozen plasma
streptokinase (Kabikinase, Streptase)	PT, PTT	• Fresh whole blood or fresh frozen plasma • Aminocaproic acid (Amicar)
urokinase (Abbokinase, Win-Kinase)	PT, PTT	• Fresh whole blood or fresh frozen plasma • Aminocaproic acid (Amicar)
warfarin (Coufarin, Coumadin, Panwarfin)	PT	• Phytonadione (vitamin K_1 [AquaMEPHYTON, Konakion, Mephyton]) • Menadiol sodium diphosphate (vitamin K_3 [Synkayvite])

Acquired Coagulation Disorders

Chronic liver disease: Associated coagulatory problems

- Circulating anticoagulants
- Disseminated intravascular coagulation
- Dysfibrinogenemia
- Excessive fibrinolytic activity
- Factor I or V deficiency
- Deficiency of vitamin K–dependent coagulation factors (II, VII, IX, and X)
- Platelet abnormalities

Intervention

The doctor will probably order parenteral vitamin K administration in the form of menadione/menadiol sodium diphosphate (vitamin K_3 [Synkayvite]) or phytonadione (vitamin K_1 [AquaMEPHYTON, Konakion, Mephyton]). To control bleeding before vitamin K takes effect (1 to 3 days), expect to give transfusions of fresh frozen plasma, which contains vitamin K–dependent proteins; these transfusions can correct bleeding immediately. If your patient has liver disease, you may need to give transfusions as often as every 4 hours. In some cases, you may also administer antifibrinolytic agents.

For a patient with a vitamin K deficiency stemming from anticoagulant therapy, the doctor may order temporary drug stoppage or antidote administration.

Nursing intervention. Take measures to control bleeding; for example, elevate the head of the bed and apply pressure.

To *prevent* vitamin K deficiency, administer vitamin K, as ordered, to newborns and to patients with malabsorption syndromes or prolonged diarrhea from colitis, Crohn's disease, or long-term antibiotic therapy. Warn the patient against self-medication with or overuse of antibiotics. If your patient's receiving an anticoagulant, carefully monitor his PT.

Self-Test

1. In the coagulation cascade, the final common pathway is triggered by which one of the following factors?
a. Factor II **b.** Factor VIII **c.** Factor X **d.** Factor XII

2. A deficiency or dysfunctioning of the plasma thromboplastin component results in which one of the following disorders?
a. Hemophilia A **b.** Hemophilia B **c.** Hemophilia C **d.** None of the above

3. When assessing a pediatric patient who may have hereditary hemorrhagic telangiectasia, it's important to remember that epistaxis is usually the first sign. True or false?
a. true **b.** false

4. Which of the following measures are appropriate for treating a patient who has immune thrombocytopenia purpura?
a. plasmapheresis and platelet transfusions **b.** plasmapheresis and prednisone **c.** prednisone and splenectomy **d.** platelet transfusions and splenectomy

5. Abnormal bleeding and a history of a hemorrhagic disorder are the hallmarks of DIC. True or false?
a. true **b.** false

6. When does parenteral vitamin K take effect?
a. after 6 to 8 hours **b.** after 12 hours **c.** after 1 to 3 days **d.** after 4 days

Answers (page numbers show where answer appears in text)
1. **c** (page 87) 2. **b** (page 91) 3. **a** (page 100) 4. **a** (page 105) 5. **b** (page 108) 6. **c** (page 115)

Lymphocyte Disorders: Lymphomas, Mononucleosis, and AIDS

Donna R. Meola, who wrote this chapter, is Assistant Director of Nursing for the department of nursing education and quality assurance at Dana Farber Cancer Institute, Boston. She received her RN diploma from St. Elizabeth Hospital and her BSN and MS from Boston College. She's also been certified by the American Association of Critical-Care Nurses.

The mononuclear phagocyte system removes worn-out cells, repairs injured tissue, and acts in both local and general body defenses. Mononuclear phagocytes include lymphocytes, monocytes, and macrophages. In this chapter, we review major lymphocyte disorders. In Chapter 8, we discuss major disorders of plasma cells (differentiated lymphocytes), monocytes, and macrophages. But first, take the time to review lymphocyte basics by reading the next few pages.

Lymphocyte development, structure, and function. Lymphocytes begin as primitive hematopoietic stem cells, which also give rise to other red and white blood cells. The stem cells that eventually become lymphocytes develop in two ways—one leading to B lymphocytes (B cells) and one leading to T lymphocytes (T cells). (See *How B and T cells mature.)*

Lymphocytes are most abundant in the bone marrow, spleen, lymph nodes, and thymus gland—the tissues where they arise. Leaving these sites, they enter the bloodstream, which carries them throughout the body; thin capillary walls allow them to pass from the blood into the interstitial fluid. From there, they eventually enter lymphatic vessels, which return them to the bloodstream. This journey takes place continuously, giving lymphocytes the best possible chance of finding and destroying any abnormal cells or foreign substances.

Based on their surface receptors' structure, lymphocytes fall into several different groups. These receptors match binding sites, known as antigenic determinants, on structurally related antigens. Thus, each lymphocyte group responds to specific types of antigens.

Functionally, lymphocytes fall into two categories:
- B cells, which differentiate into antibody-producing plasma cells
- T cells, which kill antigens directly or act in other immune responses, such as delayed hypersensitivity.

T cell subclasses can either stimulate or inhibit immune reactions. Both B and T cells can exist as long-lived memory cells.

Although B cell development isn't fully understood, animal studies indicate that B cell precursors (pre-B cells) appear in the mammalian fetal liver 3 or 4 days before B cells appear. Large lymphoid cells lacking membrane-bound antigen receptors, pre-B cells contain the IgM immunoglobulin antibody in their cytoplasm. During fetal development, these cells decrease in number in the liver while becoming more abundant in the spleen and bone marrow. Because pre-B cells appear only in the bone marrow from birth on, experts believe that B cells mature in the marrow.

Antigen receptors develop on surface membranes during B cell maturation. Secreted by the B cell, these receptors—molecules of the immunoglobulins IgM, IgD, and IgG—play a role in B cell activation.

Memory B cells permit rapid secondary (anamnestic) antibody responses, which follow reexposure to the same antigen. Regulatory B cells, which amplify or suppress lymphocyte responses, may also exist.

Continued on page 118

Lymphocyte Disorders

How B and T cells mature

Although both begin from bone marrow stem cells, B and T cells mature differently. *B cell ontogeny* was first detected in the chicken's central lymphoid organ, the bursa of Fabricius. In humans, the marrow presumably serves as the bursa equivalent; here, pre-B cells are believed to mature to B cells. These B cells then migrate to peripheral lymphoid organs, such as the lymph nodes and spleen, for storage. When an antigen-presenting cell (APC) presents an antigen to a B cell, with T cell help, the B cell is activated and proliferates. Many of these cells then differentiate into antibody-secreting plasma cells. Others remain in the lymphatic tissue as memory B cells and, upon reexposure to the same antigen, quickly differentiate into antibody-secreting plasma cells for an accelerated immune response.

In *T cell ontogeny,* T cell precursors (pre-T cells) travel to the thymus, where they mature into T cells. These T cells then leave the thymus to circulate in the blood or become constituents of the peripheral lymphoid organs.

When an APC presents an antigen in the presence of the major histocompatibility complex antigen, the T cell activates and differentiates into various subsets with overlapping functions: suppressor T cells, cytotoxic (or killer) T cells, memory T cells, lymphokine-producing T cells, and helper T cells.

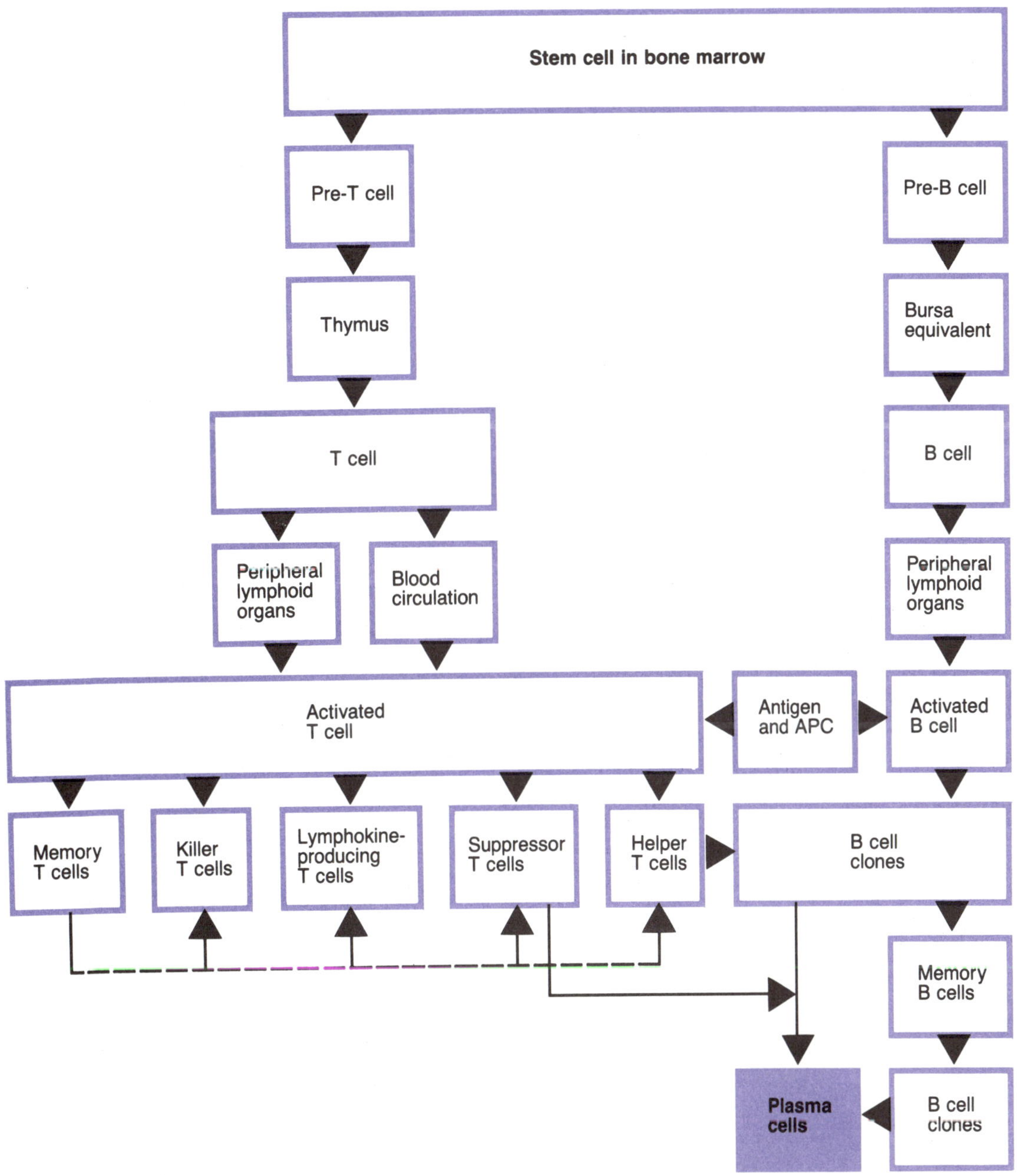

Lymphocyte Disorders

Continued

When B cells recognize an antigen, they begin to proliferate and differentiate. Proliferation increases the number of cells that can respond to the antigen. B cell growth factor, a T cell product, promotes the proliferative phase of B cell response. Differentiation changes cells into either plasma cells, which make and secrete immunoglobulins, or memory B cells, which can respond rapidly to subsequent attacks by the same antigen.

In T cell development, T cell precursors enter the thymus, where they learn to distinguish "self" from "nonself"—a process that relies on genes of the major histocompatibility complex (MHC). Many T cells die during this process; others mature and leave the thymus, traveling to peripheral lymphoid tissues.

T cell subgroups include:

- *helper T cells.* These cells stimulate B cells to proliferate and differentiate into plasma cells by recognizing both antigen determinants on B cell-bound antigens and Class II MHC molecules on antigen-presenting cells. Secreting T cells, a specific helper cell type, also help activate B cells by producing lymphokines—soluble, nonspecific immune mediators, some of which may be MHC-restricted. Secreting T cells also produce other mediators, initiate inflammatory responses, and act in delayed hypersensitivity. Without stimulation from helpers, B cells couldn't respond to many antigens. However, antigens known as thymus-independent antigens can stimulate B cells directly.
- *suppressor T cells.* These cells apparently limit the amount of T cell help available to activate B cells. This process may involve other cells as well.
- *killer (cytotoxic) T cells.* These cells kill antigens directly.
- *memory T cells.* These cells recognize antigens on reexposure and can quickly proliferate.

Besides B and T cells, a third functional lymphocyte group exists. This group includes cytotoxic cells, such as the tumor-destroying natural killer (NK) cells. How these cells recognize tumors remains a mystery, although scientists have learned that many cytotoxic cells use antibody-dependent reactions to kill their targets.

Understanding T cell subsets

Subset	Function
Killer (cytotoxic) T cells	• Produce lymphokines (cell-killing agents) • Provide delayed hypersensitivity response • Directly kill target cells for which they have an affinity
Helper T cells	• Produce lymphokines • Participate in antibody production, thereby promoting immune response
Suppressor T cells	• Regulate overall immune response
Memory T cells	• Provide immunologic memory

Lymphocyte Disorders

Lymphatic system

A network of capillaries, ducts, nodes, and organs, the lymphatic system helps preserve the body's internal fluid environment. It performs this essential task by producing, filtering, and transporting lymph and by producing various blood cells.

The lymphatic system also takes up excess fluids, fats, proteins, and other substances from body tissues and returns them to the circulation. Every 24 hours, it returns 2 to 4 liters of fluid (roughly equivalent to the total plasma volume) to the bloodstream; this fluid contains protein in an amount equal to 25% to 50% of circulating plasma protein.

Lymphatic capillaries—separate from blood-carrying capillaries—form a complex meshwork of delicate veinlike vessels that stretch to accommodate lymph. The watery extravascular fluid of tissues, lymph resembles plasma in composition but contains less protein. Thin, porous capillary walls allow large particles, such as chylomicrons, bacteria, and even blood cells, to pass through in the lymph.

Lymphatic capillaries carry lymph to the blood. Because they drain rather than perfuse or circulate fluid, they end blindly in intercellular spaces rather than forming a circuit. Capillaries exist in every tissue except bone marrow, joining to form progressively larger vessels that finally converge in two channels—the left lymphatic (thoracic) and right lymphatic ducts.

Lymphatic vessels from the body's lower half converge and empty into the cisterna chyli, a dilatation lying anterior to the vertebral column, at about the L1-L2 level. The left lymphatic duct originates from the cisterna chyli, rises along the posterior body wall, travels behind the heart, and enters the left subclavian vein near its union with the left internal jugular vein. Before entering the vein, the left lymphatic duct receives lymph vessels from the upper trunk, left arm, neck, and left side of the head. The right lymphatic duct, which enters the right subclavian vein, collects lymphatic vessels draining the right side of the head, neck, and trunk.

Unlike the circulatory system, the lymphatic system has no force to propel lymph back to the circulation. Consequently, lymphatic vessels have low pressure. Lymph moves with the help of external pressures, such as from contraction of nearby smooth or skeletal muscles and artery pulsation, along with subatmospheric intrathoracic pressure; valves prevent backflow. Smooth muscle in the walls of larger lymphatic vessels may also contribute; when lymph flow increases, this muscle becomes more active.

Lymph nodes. Before returning to the bloodstream, all lymph passes through lymph nodes, which remove foreign particles. Ranging from 1 to 15 mm in diameter, these bean-shaped structures exist at intervals along larger lymphatic vessels. Most occur in groups or chains, known by regional names. Superficial groups include the inguinal, axillary, supratrochlear, and cervical nodes. Deep groups include the mesenteric and retroperitoneal nodes. Each group receives lymph from a particular body area.

Lymph nodes have an outer covering, or capsule, of connective tissue. Inside the capsule lie an outer cortex and an inner medulla. Both consist of lymphoid tissue; the cortex also contains lymphatic nodules, or secondary follicles, containing masses of lymphocytes of various ages. Its central portion serves as a germinal center, making new lymphocytes when appropriately stimulated.

Fibrous trabeculae from the outer capsule divide the node's interior into irregular, freely communicating spaces. The reticular framework, suspended within these spaces, contains loosely meshed areas called sinusoids. Reticular cells line these structures.

Lymph enters the node via an afferent lymphatic vessel. Once inside, lymph flows through the sinusoids, where simple mechanical filtration and phagocytic cells remove bacteria, dead cells, and other foreign particles. This cleansing process proves especially important with infected lymph; the first node or group of nodes in the lymph pathway eliminates all but severe infection. After it's cleansed, lymph exits the node via efferent vessels at the hilus—a slight depression through which blood also passes.

Lymphatic organs. The lymphatic system also contains specialized lymphatic organs—the spleen, tonsils, and thymus.

Lymph node

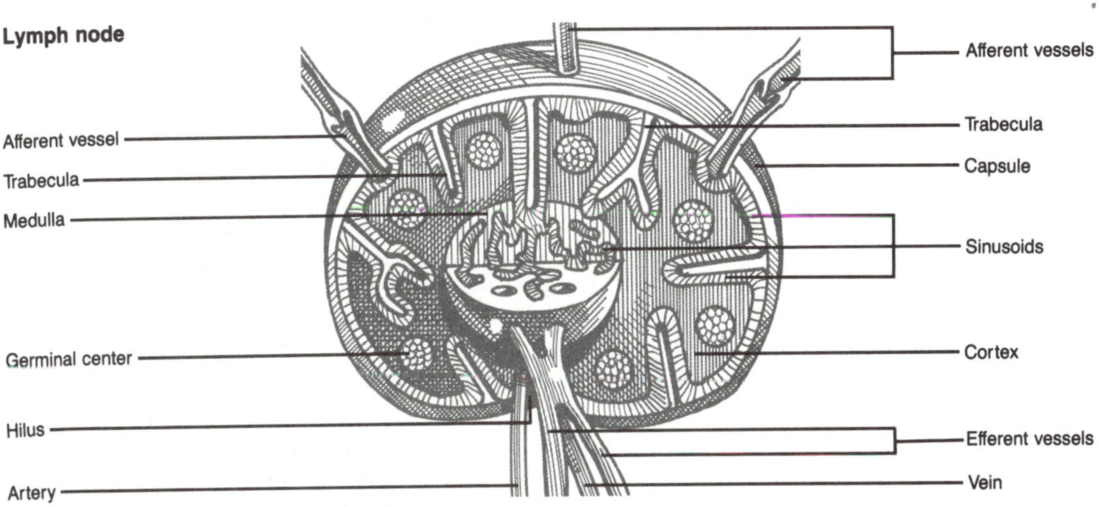

Lymphocyte Disorders

Hodgkin's disease

Hodgkin's disease: Histologic classification

- Lymphocyte predominance
- Nodular sclerosis
- Mixed cellularity
- Lymphocyte depletion

Hodgkin's disease is one of the two major lymphoma types. (For a discussion of the other type—non-Hodgkin's lymphomas—read pages 126 through 128.) Beginning as a painless, progressive lymph node enlargement, this cancer can also infiltrate the liver and spleen and may eventually spread throughout the entire body. The Reed-Sternberg cell—an abnormal, enlarged, multinucleated macrophage—proliferates uncontrollably. Along with other lymphocytes, histiocytes, eosinophils, plasma cells, and neutrophils, Reed-Sternberg cells gradually replace the normal lymph node structure.

Hodgkin's disease usually begins in one lymph node, spreading to other nodes and to the spleen through the lymphatic system. Eventually, it can travel through the bloodstream to adjacent structures. For example, because they're close to lymph nodes, the ureters and bronchi may become invaded, along with the vertebrae. Affected nodes, which grow slowly, may enlarge rapidly during fever, then revert to normal size after the fever abates.

The incidence of Hodgkin's disease peaks in two age groups—15 to 35 and 55 to 75. It's more common in men than women. A history of infectious mononucleosis, tonsillectomy, use of hydantoin derivatives (such as Dilantin), and a positive family history seem to increase the risk. Although no viral, ethnic, or immunologic factors have been conclusively identified as etiologic agents, researchers have found a familial clustering and a higher disease incidence in Hiroshima survivors.

Two classification systems—clinical staging and histologic classification—help evaluate the patient's condition. The Ann Arbor clinical staging classification, adopted in 1971, allows uniform reporting. The four stages used in this system are based on the number, location, and degree of involved nodes. (See *Staging Hodgkin's disease: Ann Arbor classification.*) Histologic classification is based on the cellular makeup of infiltrated lymph nodes. Aside from Reed-Sternberg cells, atypical giant histiocytes and other abnormal cells also appear. (See *Hodgkin's disease: Histologic classification.)*

Assessment

The most common sign of Hodgkin's disease is an enlarged, painless cervical lymph node. Other signs and symptoms stem from two main causes: pressure from enlarged nodes on nearby structures and disease infiltration into vital organs. (For example, nodal compression of a ureter may cause hydronephrosis.)

When taking your patient's medical history, ask yourself the following questions:

- Has the patient had a recent upper respiratory or other infection? (Defective cell-mediated immunity commonly accompanies Hodgkin's disease.) The more severe the disease, the greater the susceptibility to infection. A patient with advanced disease usually suffers repeated bacterial, viral, fungal, and parasitic infections from pancytopenia. In a few cases, respiratory symptoms result from mediastinal involvement.
- Has the patient had fever or night sweats? Has he suffered from anorexia or experienced unexplained weight loss? These nonspecific

Continued on page 122

Lymphocyte Disorders

Staging Hodgkin's disease: Ann Arbor classification

The Ann Arbor classification system divides Hodgkin's disease into four stages. In Stage I, the disease resides in a single lymph node region (I) or a single extralymphatic organ (I_E). In Stage II, the disease appears in two or more nodes on the same side of the diaphragm (II) and in an extralymphatic organ (II_E) or the spleen (II_S). Stage III indicates disease on both sides of the diaphragm (III) and perhaps in an extralymphatic organ (III_E), the spleen (III_S), or both. Stage IV describes diffuse or disseminated involvement of one or more extralymphatic organs or tissues, with or without associated lymph node involvement. Each stage can be further divided into Category A, for patients without defined symptoms, and Category B, for patients with such defined symptoms as recent unexplained weight loss, fever, and night sweats.

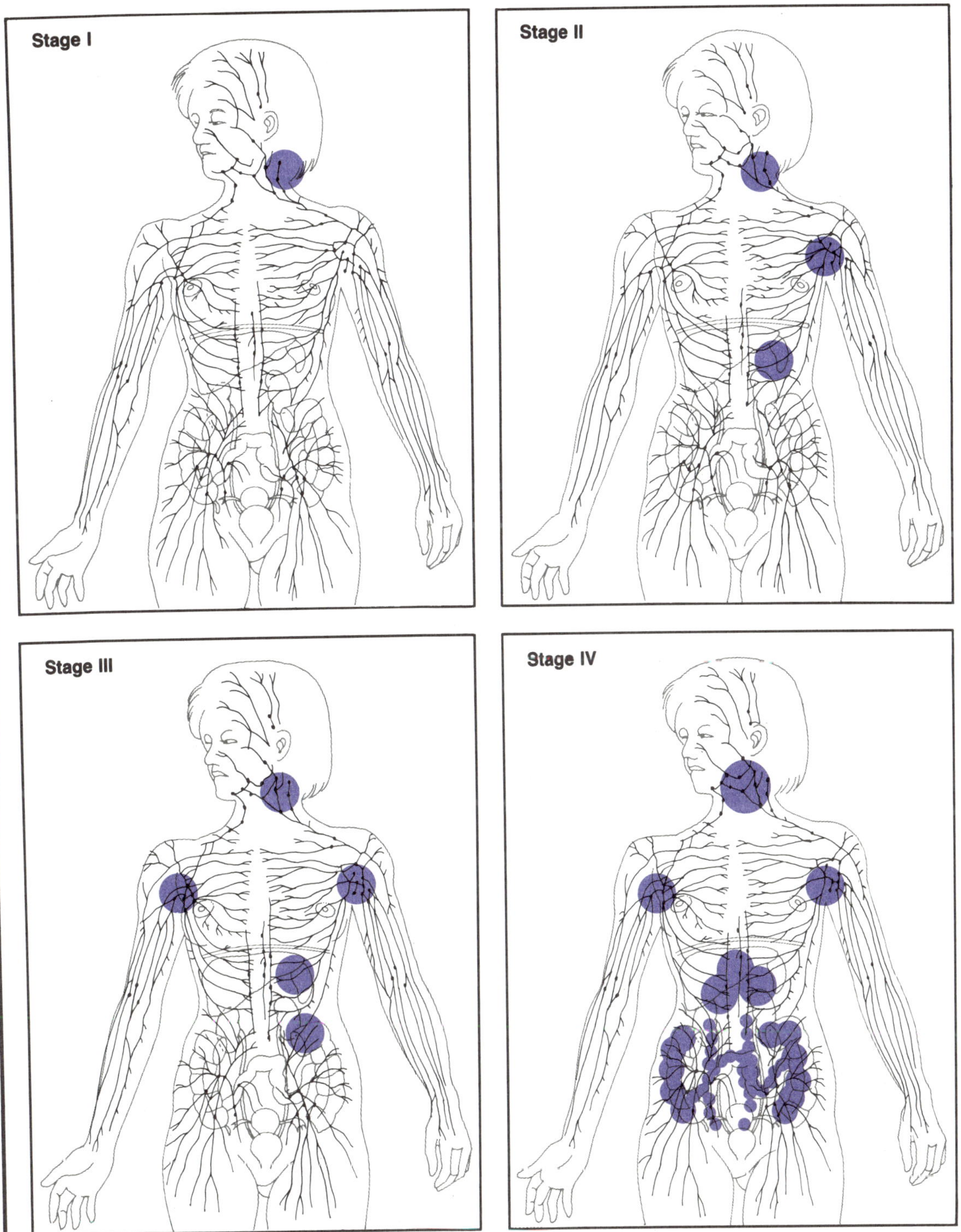

Lymphocyte Disorders

Lymph node biopsy: Suggestive findings

These enlarged, abnormal histiocytes (Reed-Sternberg cells) from an excised lymph node suggest Hodgkin's disease. Note the large, distinct nucleoli. Reed-Sternberg cells indicate Hodgkin's disease when they coexist with one of these four histologic patterns: lymphocyte predominance, mixed cellularity, lymphocyte depletion, or nodular sclerosis.

Reed-Sternberg cells

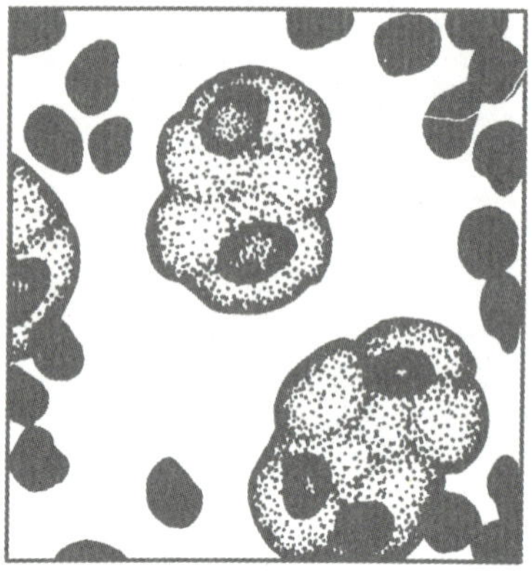

Hodgkin's disease—*continued*

symptoms commonly arise in older patients. Rarely, a patient has the Pel-Ebstein fever pattern, in which several days of intermittent fever alternate with afebrile periods.

- Does the patient complain of dysphagia, nausea, vomiting, or abdominal fullness? Esophageal or bowel obstruction from enlarged abdominal lymph nodes causes these problems.
- Does the patient have a persistent cough or dypsnea? These symptoms result from tracheal compression by enlarged nodes.
- Does he suffer from paresthesias or lower extremity weakness? These problems usually signal spinal cord compression by vertebral bone involvement and subsequent tumor growth.
- Does he have progressive dyspnea, cough, and orthopnea? These signs and symptoms, which indicate superior vena cava syndrome, stem from superior vena cava compression by enlarged nodes. As central venous pressure increases, the patient may complain of headache, vertigo, and drowsiness. Eventually, he may become stuporous and lose consciousness. *Important:* Compression of the superior vena cava, trachea, or spinal cord are medical emergencies. Notify the doctor immediately to prevent permanent disability or death.
- Does the patient have pruritus? An early sign of Hodgkin's disease, pruritus may be mild at first, then worsen as the disease progresses.
- Does the patient complain of pain? If so, where? Although rare, localized pain—usually in the throat, epigastric area, or other regions near enlarged lymph nodes—may occur after drinking alcohol. Nerve pain may arise in advanced disease stages.
- Does the patient look jaundiced or anemic? These signs may appear in late disease stages from liver involvement or red blood cell hemolysis.
- Does the patient complain of urinary disturbances or flank pain? These problems suggest ureteral compression by enlarged nodes, possibly leading to renal failure.

During the physical examination, inspect and palpate all lymph nodes. Note their size, consistency (hard or soft), and whether they're fixed or movable, tender or painless. Because nodes on the left side are more commonly affected than those on the right, the disease can spread to the abdomen via the thoracic duct.

Inspect the patient's face, neck, and upper torso for edema and check for chest and abdominal collateral vein distention; these signs may indicate superior vena cava syndrome. Ascites, dependent and periorbital edema, pleural effusion, pallor, and orthostatic hypotension may mean renal failure. (*Note:* Massive edema, accompanied by proteinuria and hypoalbuminemia, suggests nephrotic syndrome, which may precede Hodgkin's disease by several months.)

Palpate the patient's abdomen—especially the liver and spleen—noting any abdominal masses (possibly from enlarged abdominal nodes) and liver involvement. If you suspect liver involvement, assess the patient for jaundice and signs of liver failure (including ascites, level of consciousness changes, peripheral edema, and jaundice).

Lymphocyte Disorders

In rare cases, patients may have lymphomatous lesions outside the lymphatic tissue—especially in the breasts and testicles—so be sure to palpate for masses in these areas. Also note any bone tenderness.

Diagnostic studies. The doctor must rule out other disorders that cause enlarged lymph nodes, such as cytomegalovirus infection, leukemia, and systemic lupus erythematosus. Hematologic tests may show mild to severe normocytic anemia; normochromic anemia; elevated, normal, or reduced white blood cell count and differential showing any combination of neutrophilia, lymphocytopenia, monocytosis, and eosinophilia. Elevated serum alkaline phosphatase indicates liver or bone involvement. The patient with kidney involvement may have an elevated blood urea nitrogen level.

Expect the doctor to order a lymph node biopsy to check for Reed-Sternberg cells; bone marrow, liver, and spleen biopsies; and chest X-ray, abdominal computed tomography (CT) scan, and a bone scan to assess lymph node and organ involvement.

A few patients may show a mediastinal or hilar mass on X-ray. If these patients don't have enlarged peripheral nodes, the doctor will probably order a lung CT scan to identify other involved nodes. Mediastinoscopy may be necessary to determine mediastinal node involvement. X-rays of the vertebrae, pelvis, proximal long bones, and areas of bony tenderness help determine involvement in these areas.

For a symptomatic patient showing no peripheral node enlargement and a normal chest X-ray, expect the doctor to order bilateral pedal lymphangiography. This test reveals inguinal, iliac, and paraaortic nodes within 24 hours of dye injection. Monitor your patient closely if he has respiratory disease because the dye used in the test can exacerbate his condition.

Diagnostic tests also allow disease staging. A staging laparotomy will be performed if the patient's under age 55 or lacks obvious Stage III or IV disease, lymphocyte predominance subtype histology, or medical contraindications.

Planning

Focus your nursing care on promoting patient comfort, offering emotional support, maintaining optimal nutritional status and fluid and electrolyte balance, and teaching the patient about the disease.

Nursing diagnoses. Before determining your nursing care plan, develop the nursing diagnosis by identifying the patient's actual or potential problem, then relating it to its cause. Possible nursing diagnoses for a patient with Hodgkin's disease include the following:

- activity intolerance; related to fatigue resulting from decreased blood or tissue oxygenation
- injury, potential for (bleeding); related to treatment-induced platelet level reduction
- nutrition, alteration in (less than body requirements); related to increased metabolism secondary to cancer cell proliferation
- skin integrity, impairment of (potential); related to radiation therapy

Continued on page 124

Lymphocyte Disorders

Sample nursing care plan: Hodgkin's disease

Nursing diagnosis	Expected outcomes
Body image, disturbance in; related to alopecia	The patient will: • acknowledge that he's losing his hair. • verbalize his feelings about losing his hair. • participate in decisions about hair and scalp care.
Nursing interventions	**Discharge planning**
• Inform patient that hair loss usually begins 2 to 3 weeks after radiation therapy starts. Warn him that his hair roots may hurt before his hair begins falling out. • If hair loss will be temporary (as after radiation therapy of 1,500 to 3,000 rads), reassure patient that his hair will probably grow back within 1 to 3 months after therapy ends. Explain that new hair may be a different color, texture, and/or thickness. • If the patient will receive radiation doses of 4,500 rads or more, warn him that hair loss will probably be permanent. (*Note:* Doses between 3,000 and 4,500 rads cause permanent hair loss in some patients.) • For patient with anticipated partial hair loss or thinning, explain ways to minimize loss. For example, advise him to brush and comb hair gently; wash hair only when necessary and avoid harsh shampoo, cream rinse, and other hair products; and avoid hair dryers, curling irons, curlers, hair clips, rubber bands, or other constrictive devices. • Encourage patient to use a wig, toupee, scarf, or other head covering. Advise him to try on a wig or toupee before hair loss begins, to ease adjustment.	• Review hair and scalp care with patient; answer any questions he might have. • Advise him to contact the American Cancer Society for advice on wigs, if necessary. • Remind the patient to wear a hat, scarf, or turban if a wig or toupee becomes too uncomfortable. • Refer patient and family to a support group, such as One Day at a Time. • Consult with a psychiatric nurse specialist and community health nurse to provide continuing emotional support at home, as necessary.

Hodgkins's disease—*continued*

• infection, potential for; related to increased production of immature white blood cells
• body image, disturbance in; related to alopecia
• knowledge deficit; related to prognosis and treatment
• comfort, alteration in (pain); related to pressure from or infiltration of lymphoma on vital organs.

The sample nursing care plan above shows expected outcomes, nursing interventions, and discharge planning for one nursing diagnosis listed above. However, you'll want to tailor each care plan to fit your patient's needs.

Intervention

Depending on the disease's extent, histologic classification, and clinical staging, the doctor will order chemotherapy, radiation therapy, or both. Appropriate treatment permits longer survival and may even provide a cure.

A patient with Stage I or II disease requires only radiation therapy, whereas a patient with Stage III disease will probably need both radiation and chemotherapy. For Stage IV disease, expect the doctor to order chemotherapy alone, which sometimes induces a complete

Lymphocyte Disorders

remission. Chemotherapy can be given in various combinations of mechlorethamine (Mustargen), vincristine (Oncovin), procarbazine (Matulane), prednisone (such as Deltasone or Orasone), cyclophosphamide (Cytoxan), vinblastine (Velban), carmustine (BCNU [BiCNU]), bleomycin (Blenoxane), doxorubicin (Adriamycin), and dacarbazine (DTIC). The MOPP protocol (mechlorethamine, Oncovin, procarbazine, and prednisone)—known as the gold standard—was the first combination to cure patients with generalized Hodgkin's disease. ABVD (Adriamycin, bleomycin, vinblastine, and dacarbazine)—another useful combination—may be given six times at 28-day intervals. A patient receiving these drugs may need antiemetics, sedatives, or antidiarrheals to alleviate adverse gastrointestinal effects.

Therapy based on careful staging and intensive use of radiation, either alone or with chemotherapy, has achieved a 90% long-term survival rate. Patients with Stage I or II disease who receive intensive radiation therapy have the best prognosis; Stage III patients who receive MOPP chemotherapy, alone or with radiation therapy, have a survival rate that's almost as favorable. Stage IV patients have a slightly worse prognosis, with a 5-year survival rate approaching 40%. Patients over age 40 have a poorer prognosis than younger patients, as do those who seek medical care only after suffering fever, weight loss, and night sweats.

Nursing intervention. The patient with Hodgkin's disease, who typically has a history of good health, may be especially anxious and fearful. Be sure to provide emotional support and, if necessary, refer him for counseling. Ease his anxiety by sharing your optimism

Continued on page 126

Radiation therapy: Identifying and managing adverse effects

Irradiated region	Possible adverse effect	Nursing actions
Abdomen	Nausea	Eliminate foods patient can't tolerate (seeing and smelling them could trigger or exacerbate nausea).
	Vomiting	Administer antiemetic, as ordered; monitor fluid and electrolyte levels.
Chest	Esophagitis	Serve puréed foods; administer antacid, diphenhydramine, lidocaine, xylocaine viscous solution, and/or antiemetics, as ordered.
	Nausea	See "Abdomen," above.
	Pneumonitis	Administer oxygen and steroids, as ordered; encourage fluid intake.
Head and neck	Dry mouth	Provide fluids, mouth spray, or artificial saliva to keep mucous membranes moist.
Pelvis	Diarrhea	Serve low-fiber diet; give antidiarrheal medication, as ordered.
	Cystitis	Encourage intake of 3,000 ml fluid/day (unless contraindicated); tell patient to avoid spicy foods, alcohol, coffee, and tea.
Scalp (whole brain)	Alopecia	Tell patient to avoid excessive shampooing, hair dryers, sun, cold, and heat.

Note: Radiation exposure on any body region can lead to erythema and dry and wet skin desquamation. To minimize these effects, teach the patient to avoid soaps, lotions, perfume, heat, sun, and irritating fabrics. Use tepid water with peroxide or saline solution when providing skin care or bathing the patient.

Lymphocyte Disorders

Hodgkins's disease—*continued*

about his prognosis. Advise him and his family that they can obtain information and supportive counseling from the local chapter of the American Cancer Association or from local support groups such as One Day at a Time.

Teach your patient about the adverse effects of chemotherapy and/or radiation therapy and provide written material explaining how to care for himself while undergoing therapy. Because radiation and chemotherapy can cause alopecia, prepare him for this possibility. Tell an outpatient receiving radiation or chemotherapy to observe these precautions:

- Watch for and report adverse effects of radiation and chemotherapy, particularly anorexia, nausea, vomiting, diarrhea, and menstrual irregularity (which may or may not be permanent).
- Minimize adverse effects by maintaining good nutrition (promoted by eating frequent small meals that include favorite foods); drinking plenty of fluids; pacing activities to counteract chemotherapy-induced fatigue; and keeping skin on irradiated areas dry.
- Control pain and bleeding from stomatitis by using a soft toothbrush, cotton swab, or anesthetic mouthwash, such as lidocaine (as prescribed); applying petrolatum to the lips; and avoiding astringent mouthwashes.
- If the patient is male, he may want to deposit sperm in a sperm bank.
- If the patient is female and of childbearing age, advise her to delay pregnancy until prolonged remission, since chemotherapy and radiation therapy may cause genetic mutations and spontaneous abortions.

Evaluation

Base your evaluation on the expected outcomes listed on the nursing care plan. To determine whether your patient has improved, ask yourself such questions as these:

- Does the patient acknowledge his alopecia?
- Does he talk about how it feels to lose his hair?
- Does he make decisions regarding hair and scalp care?

The answers to these questions will help you evaluate your patient's status and the effectiveness of his care. Keep in mind that these questions stem from the sample care plan on page 124. Your questions may differ.

Other lymphomas

Non-Hodgkin's lymphomas

Also known as lymphosarcomas, non-Hodgkin's lymphomas are characterized by proliferation of lymphoid cells other than Reed-Sternberg cells. Such lymphomas may arise in the lymph nodes, spleen, Waldeyer's ring (lymphatic tissue encircling the nasopharynx and oropharynx), bone marrow, or GI tract. The disease may remain localized for years or it may involve several lymph nodes from the start, then spread to the bone marrow, liver, lungs, and

Non-Hodgkin's lymphomas: Rappaport classification

Nodular
- Lymphocytic, poorly differentiated
- Mixed lymphocytic-histiocytic
- Histiocytic

Diffuse
- Lymphocytic, well differentiated
- Lymphocytic, poorly differentiated
- Mixed lymphocytic-histiocytic
- Undifferentiated
- Histiocytic

Lymphocyte Disorders

Burkitt's lymphoma

Composed of undifferentiated lymphoreticular cells, Burkitt's lymphoma most commonly affects children. Typically, the abnormal cells form a large lesion in the jaw. As the disease progresses, it may involve organs above and below the diaphragm, usually the kidneys or gonads. Advanced disease involves the bone marrow and/or central nervous system.

Rare in the United States, Burkitt's lymphoma appears most commonly in Central Africa. Climatic factors seem to determine its distribution, suggesting an infectious agent and insect vector as etiologic agents. Strong evidence points to the Epstein-Barr virus as the cause.

Burkitt's lymphoma is highly curable—even in advanced stages—with cyclophosphamide (Cytoxan, Neosar). High intermittent doses of this drug produce long-term disease-free survival in about 70% to 80% of Stage I and II patients and in about 30% of Stage III patients. If the patient has widespread Burkitt's lymphoma, the doctor will use a cautious treatment approach—rapid tumor destruction can cause hyperkalemia, hyperphosphatemia, and hypocalcemia, which may produce fatal cardiac dysrhythmias. Hyperuricemia leading to acute renal failure may also occur.

Lymphoblastic lymphoma

Among the most common non-Hodgkin's lymphomas in children, undifferentiated lymphoblastic lymphoma consists of many cells containing lymphoblasts. Resembling acute lymphocytic leukemia (ALL), this diffuse, highly aggressive tumor typically occurs in older children as well as in young adults. Patients usually seek medical help for signs and symptoms associated with an anterior mediastinal mass.

Treatment usually includes combination chemotherapy and radiation therapy. Despite aggressive therapy, however, patients have a poor prognosis; the disease usually spreads rapidly to the bone marrow, peripheral blood vessels, and meninges.

other organs. Non-Hodgkin's lymphomas more frequently involve nonlymphatic tissue than does Hodgkin's disease.

Non-Hodgkin's lymphomas can be classified by several different systems, based on tumor histology, cytology, and immunologic features. Experts disagree, however, as to the relative usefulness and accuracy of these systems and have yet to settle on a standard nomenclature. For clinical purposes, the Rappaport classification system may prove most useful and reliable. (See *Non-Hodgkin's lymphomas: Rappaport classification.*)

Nodularity ranks as the most important histologic distinction among non-Hodgkin's lymphomas. Its presence predicts prolonged survival; most diffuse lymphomas, in contrast, carry a poor survival rate. Diffuse, well–differentiated lymphocytic lymphoma is an exception; patients with this disease have a median survival rate greater than 5 years. Representing the tissue manifestation of chronic lymphocytic leukemia, this lymphoma sometimes precedes leukemia by months or even years. Lymphomas with a histiocytic histology carry a worse prognosis. Like Hodgkin's disease, non-Hodgkin's lymphomas have an unknown etiology. Some experts suspect that a viral agent may be responsible. Up to 8,000 new cases appear in the United States each year. Two to three times more common in males than in females, these cancers rise in incidence with age (median age is 50). However, they occur in all age groups. Although rare in children, they're one to three times more common and cause twice as many deaths as Hodgkin's disease in children under age 15. Whites, especially those of Jewish ancestry, have a higher incidence than nonwhites.

Assessment. Although many patients respond well to treatment, they're less likely to achieve long remissions or cures compared with patients who have Hodgkin's disease. The patient with non-Hodgkin's lymphoma typically reports enlarged, painless lymph nodes (especially in the cervical and supraclavicular areas), perhaps accompanied by enlarged tonsils and adenoids. He may also complain of back pain, from enlarged retroperitoneal nodes (which can also cause ascites). Ask him if he's had fever, night sweats, anorexia, weight loss, or pruritus—systemic signs that can appear long before the lymphoma becomes apparent. Find out if he's suffered recent fractures, a possible indication of bone lesions, or GI problems, which may result from bowel lesions and subsequent ulcerative disease and malabsorption. Occasionally, nephrotic syndrome accompanies malignant lymphomas and may precede diagnosis by several months. A history of headache or visual problems, including diplopia and photophobia, may signal meningeal lesions.

When performing the physical examination, inspect and palpate the patient's lymph nodes. Check for jaundice, indicating bile duct compression from nodal enlargement in the porta hepatis. Also check for soft-tissue masses, nuchal rigidity, peripheral edema of the legs and perineum or scrotum, and pleural effusions (from hilar adenopathy or lymphomatous pleural involvement).

Assess for signs of hydronephrosis, bowel obstruction, paralysis (with advanced disease), and superior vena cava and spinal cord compression.

Continued on page 128

Lymphocyte Disorders

Other lymphomas—*continued*

Diagnostic tests. Diagnosis requires histologic evaluation of biopsied lymph nodes, tonsils, bone marrow, liver, bowel, skin, or, if necessary, of tissue removed during exploratory laparotomy. This evaluation distinguishes non-Hodgkin's lymphoma from Hodgkin's disease.

Other relevant tests include bone and chest X-rays, lymphangiography, liver and spleen scan, abdominal CT scan, and excretory urography. The doctor will also order various laboratory tests, including complete blood count (which may show anemia), uric acid (elevated or normal), serum calcium level (elevated if bone lesions are present), serum protein level (normal), and liver function studies.

Intervention. Radiation therapy and cytotoxic chemotherapy have proven effective against non-Hodgkin's lymphoma. A patient with early, localized disease may receive radiation; whole-body radiation helps cure tumors with nodular or diffuse histologies.

For some patients, the doctor will order combination chemotherapy for maximum effectiveness. Cyclophosphamide, vincristine, and prednisone have induced complete remission in about 70% to 80% of patients with nodular histology and about 20% to 55% of those with diffuse histology. Other combinations—such as BACOP (bleomycin [Blenoxane], doxorubicin [Adriamycin], cyclophosphamide [Cytoxan], vincristine [Oncovin], and prednisone)—have induced prolonged remission and even cures in patients with diffuse histology.

Nursing intervention. Like Hodgkin's disease, non-Hodgkin's lymphoma calls for nursing measures aimed at helping the patient cope with adverse treatment effects and providing emotional support. For example:

- Observe for anorexia, nausea, vomiting, and diarrhea. Consult with the dietitian to plan frequent small meals that include the patient's favorite foods. Schedule meals around treatment.
- If the patient can't tolerate oral feedings, administer I.V. fluids and, if necessary, give antiemetics and sedatives, as ordered.
- Instruct the patient to keep irradiated skin dry.
- Provide emotional support by listening to the patient's concerns. Teach him and his family about the diagnosis and prognosis. If needed, refer them to the local chapter of the American Cancer Society or a local support group for information and counseling. Stress the need for continued treatment and follow-up care.

Mycosis fungoides

A rare, chronic, malignant T cell lymphoma of unknown cause, mycosis fungoides (MF) originates in the skin, eventually affecting lymph nodes and internal organs. Usually, it begins as an itchy red rash. Months or even years later, plaques and lymphomatous tumors infiltrate the skin. The resulting mushroom–like growths, varying from 1 to 5 cm (0.4" to 2") in diameter, may cover the entire body, causing discomfort and disfigurement.

MF strikes more than 1,000 Americans each year. It occurs in all races and affects men more often than women. Onset usually occurs

Angioimmunoblastic lymphadenopathy

A newly described disorder of unknown cause, angioimmunoblastic (immunoblastic) lymphadenopathy resembles lymphoma (although it's considered nonneoplastic). It produces generalized adenopathy, liver and spleen enlargement, maculopapular rash, night sweats, fever, and weight loss. Laboratory evaluation commonly reveals hemolytic anemia, polyclonal hypergammaglobulinemia, or both. Affected nodes show abnormal architecture with infiltration by lymphocytes, immunoblasts, plasma cells, and eosinophils. Small capillary proliferation and deposition of amorphous interstitial material also occur. In some cases, the disease progresses to immunoblastic sarcoma.

Treatment—usually combination chemotherapy or radiation therapy—typically proves ineffective. Most patients die within 1 or 2 years of diagnosis.

Autologous bone marrow transplant

This experimental procedure may offer hope for adults with relapsed non-Hodgkin's lymphoma. First, the doctor removes a bone marrow specimen. The patient then receives high-dose chemotherapy and total–body radiation to kill cancer cells. After the extracted marrow has been cleaned of these cells by anti-B1 monoclonal antibodies, the marrow's reinfused into the patient.

Studies reveal that autologous bone marrow transplants prove most effective in patients with small tumors who still respond to conventional chemotherapy. Potentially, the procedure could help 5,000 to 10,000 patients each year. However, it's expensive and highly toxic. Many experts believe that the procedure needs further study and refinement before it can be used extensively.

Lymphocyte Disorders

after age 40. MF patients have an average life expectancy of 7 to 10 years after diagnosis. If correctly treated—particularly before it spreads past the skin—MF may remain in remission for years. However, once the disease reaches the tumor stage, it quickly progresses to severe disability or death.

Although the etiology of MF is unknown, it may have environmental, genetic, and infectious roots. The patient may have a history of exposure to certain drugs or toxic substances, perhaps from working in a plant that produces machinery, petrochemicals, metals, or textiles. MF may be familial, since reports indicate that more than one family may have MF or MF combined with other lymphomas and leukemias.

Assessment. The patient will report pruritus and rashes. Look for generalized erythroderma; infiltrated, thickened, or scaly skin patches; tumors; and ulcerations.

Extracutaneous disease often manifests as pulmonary lesions, including infiltrates, nodules, pleural effusion, mediastinal adenopathy, or hilar adenopathy. Other lesions may appear in the bones, eyes, kidneys, liver, bone marrow, oral cavity, upper respiratory tract, cardiovascular system, GI tract, and central nervous system.

Diagnostic tests. A clear diagnosis relies on a history of multiple, varied, and progressively severe skin lesions and on characteristic histologic evidence of lymphoma cell infiltration of the skin. Lymph nodes and visceral organs may be involved. MF may escape diagnosis until the skin contains sufficient lymphoma cells to show up in biopsy.

Other confirming tests include complete blood count and differential; a finger stick smear for Sézary cells (abnormal circulating lymphocytes), which may be present in erythrodermic MF variants (Sézary syndrome); blood chemistry tests to screen for visceral dysfunction; chest X-ray; liver and spleen scanning; lymphangiography; and lymph node biopsy to assess histologic involvement. These tests also help stage the disease—a necessary prerequisite to treatment.

Intervention. Treatment depends on several factors, including disease stage and progression rate, previous treatment and results, the patient's age and overall health, and available treatment facilities. Treatment options include:

- topical, intralesional, or systemic corticosteroid therapy
- phototherapy
- methoxsalen (Oxsoralen) photochemotherapy
- radiation therapy
- topical, intralesional, or systemic mechlorethamine (Mustargen)
- other systemic chemotherapy.

Expect the doctor to order topical mechlorethamine to induce remission in a patient with pretumorous MF. As ordered, administer preliminary I.V. infusions of small Mustargen doses before beginning topical treatment (although the value of this practice remains unproven, it presumably helps reduce the risk of allergic sensitization).

Continued on page 130

Combination chemotherapy: Four regimens

For a patient with non-Hodgkin's lymphoma, the doctor may order one of the following combination chemotherapy regimens:

CVP (repeated every 3 weeks as tolerated)
- cyclophosphamide (Cytoxan, Neosar)
- vincristine (Oncovin)
- prednisone (Deltasone, Orasone)

COPP (repeated every 4 weeks as tolerated)
- cyclophosphamide
- vincristine (Oncovin)
- procarbazine (Matulane)
- prednisone

CHOP (repeated every 3 to 4 weeks as tolerated)
- cyclophosphamide
- doxorubicin (Adriamycin)
- vincristine (Oncovin)
- prednisone

BACOP (repeated every 4 weeks as tolerated)
- bleomycin (Blenoxane)
- doxorubicin (Adriamycin)
- cyclophosphamide
- vincristine (Oncovin)
- prednisone

Staging mycosis fungoides

Skin involvement (T):
T_0 Clinically or histopathologically suspicious lesions
T_1 Premycotic lesions, papules, or plaques involving less than 10% of the skin surface
T_2 Premycotic lesions, papules, or plaques involving more than 10% of the skin surface
T_3 One or more skin tumors
T_4 Extensive, often generalized erythroderma

Peripheral lymph node status (N):
N_0 Clinically normal; no pathologic involvement
N_1 Clinically abnormal; no pathologic involvement
N_2 Clinically normal; pathologic involvement
N_3 Clinically abnormal; pathologic involvement

Visceral organ status (M):
M_0 No pathologic involvement
M_1 Pathologic involvement

Lymphocyte Disorders

Other lymphomas—*continued*

Total-body electron beam radiation, less toxic to internal organs than standard photon beam radiation, has induced remission in some patients with early-stage MF.

Most patients with advanced MF will receive chemotherapy involving such agents as cyclophosphamide, chlorambucil (Leukeran), methotrexate (with or without folinic acid rescue), doxorubicin, vincristine, or bleomycin.

Nursing intervention. Focus your nursing care on these measures:
- If the patient has trouble applying Mustargen to all skin surfaces, give assistance (be sure to wear gloves to prevent contact sensitization).
- If the patient's receiving drug treatment, report adverse effects—particularly infection—immediately.
- If the patient's receiving chemotherapy or radiation to the head, he'll probably experience alopecia. Wearing a wig or toupee may boost his self-image until his hair grows back; recommend or give medicated oil baths to ease erythema.
- Because pruritus commonly worsens at night, administer larger bedtime doses of antipruritics or sedatives, as ordered and needed, to ensure a good night's sleep. If the patient has had difficulty sleeping, postpone early-morning care to give him more rest.
- The patient with pruritus has an overwhelming need to scratch—possibly to the point of removing epidermis and replacing pruritus with pain, which he may find more tolerable. Realize that you can't keep such a patient from scratching but can help minimize the damage. Advise the patient to keep his fingernails short and clean and to wear white cotton gloves when itching becomes unbearable.
- Malignant skin lesions can make the patient depressed, fearful, and self-conscious. Explain the disease and its stages to help the patient and family understand and accept it. Provide reassurance and support by demonstrating a positive but realistic attitude. Reinforce your verbal support by touching the patient without any hint of anxiety or distaste.

Infectious mononucleosis: Microscopic findings

Large, reactive lymphocytes interspersed with normal erythrocytes, such as those shown here, characterize infectious mononucleosis.

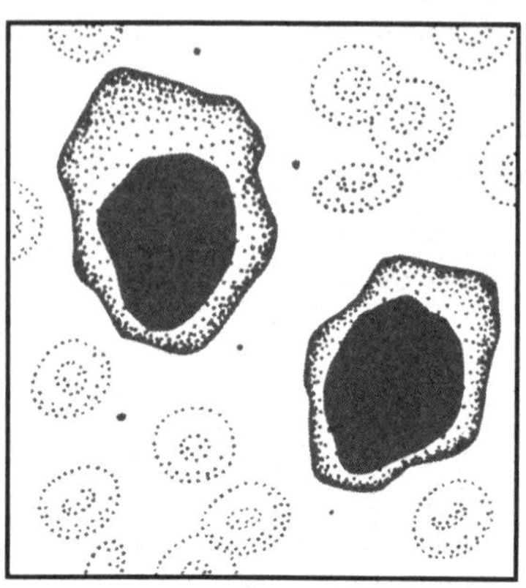

Infectious mononucleosis

An acute disease, infectious mononucleosis is caused by the Epstein-Barr virus (EBV), a member of the herpes group. Its hallmarks include fever, sore throat, and cervical lymphadenopathy. Fairly common in the United States, Canada, and Europe, the disease primarily affects young adults and children, although children usually get a mild version that's easily overlooked. Both sexes are equally susceptible. College students usually contract the disease in the early spring or early fall, a seasonal variation not found among the general population.

The disease probably spreads by the oral-pharyngeal route: most patients carry EBV in the throat during the acute infection and for an indefinite period afterward. It can also spread by blood transfusion and has appeared after cardiac surgery as "post-pump perfusion" syndrome. The contagious period probably starts before symptoms develop and lasts until the fever subsides and oral-pharyngeal lesions disappear. Patients have an excellent prognosis,

Lymphocyte Disorders

although a few major complications develop, such as splenic rupture, aseptic meningitis, encephalitis, hemolytic anemia, and Guillain-Barré syndrome.

Assessment

Signs and symptoms of infectious mononucleosis mimic those of many other infectious diseases. After an incubation period of about 10 days in children and 30 to 50 days in adults, prodromal symptoms appear—headache, malaise, and fatigue. After 3 to 5 days, patients typically develop a classic symptom triad: sore throat, cervical lymphadenopathy, and temperature fluctuation, with an evening peak of 101° to 102° F. (38.3° to 38.9° C.). Splenomegaly, hepatomegaly, stomatitis, exudative tonsillitis, or pharyngitis may also develop. Symptoms usually subside about 6 to 10 days after disease onset but may persist for weeks.

When taking your patient's history, ask him whether he's recently experienced sore throat, fever, malaise, fatigue, or headache. During the physical examination, look for a maculopapular rash (resembling rubella), inspect his mouth for stomatitis, and check for a reddened throat. You may also detect lymphadenopathy and jaundice.

Diagnostic tests. These laboratory findings confirm infectious mononucleosis:

- white blood cell (WBC) count increased 10,000 to 20,000/μl during the 2nd and 3rd weeks of illness. Lymphocytes and monocytes account for 50% to 70% of the total WBC count; more than 20% of lymphocytes are atypical.
- heterophil antibodies (agglutinins for sheep RBCs) in serum, drawn during the acute illness and at 3- to 4-week intervals, increased to about four times normal.
- indirect immunofluorescence showing antibodies to EBV and cellular antigens. Such testing's usually more definitive than heterophil antibody findings.
- abnormal liver function studies.

Planning

Focus your nursing care on teaching the patient and his family about the need for rest and adequate nutrition, and urge them to watch for and report signs and symptoms of complications.

Nursing diagnoses. Before determining your nursing care plan, develop the nursing diagnosis by identifying the patient's actual or potential problem, then relating it to its cause. Possible nursing diagnoses for the patient with infectious mononucleosis include:

- knowledge deficit; related to need for long-term rest
- social isolation; related to long-term rest
- coping, ineffective (individual); related to social isolation
- communication, impaired (verbal); related to pharyngitis
- diversional activity, deficit; related to fatigue and malaise
- comfort, alteration in (pain); related to headache
- oral mucous membrane, alteration in; related to stomatitis and tonsillitis
- nutrition, alteration in (less than body requirements); related to fatigue and malaise
- self-care deficit (bathing/hygiene); related to fatigue and malaise.

Continued on page 132

Lymphocyte Disorders

Infectious mononucleosis—*continued*

The sample nursing care plan below shows expected outcomes, nursing interventions, and discharge planning for one nursing diagnosis listed above. However, you'll want to tailor each care plan to fit your patient's needs.

Intervention

Because infectious mononucleosis resists antimicrobial treatment, therapy's essentially supportive: symptomatic relief, bed rest during the acute febrile period, and aspirin or another analgesic for headache and sore throat. If severe throat inflammation causes airway obstruction, the doctor will probably order steroids to reduce swelling and avoid tracheotomy. Splenic rupture, marked by sudden abdominal pain, warrants splenectomy. About 20% of patients also have streptococcal pharyngotonsillitis and should receive antibiotic therapy for at least 10 days.

Nursing intervention. Nursing measures for the patient with infectious mononucleosis include the following:

- Because uncomplicated infectious mononucleosis doesn't require hospitalization, be sure to teach your patient about the disease. Explain that convalescence may take several weeks or even months, usually until the WBC count returns to normal. Stress the need for bed rest during the acute period. If the patient's a student, tell him he may continue less demanding school assignments and see his friends but should avoid long, difficult projects until after recovery. Also advise him to avoid excessive physical activity to prevent splenic rupture.
- To help combat depression caused by chronic fatigue and malaise, offer emotional support.
- To help relieve throat pain, advise the patient to drink milk shakes, fruit juices, and broths; eat cool, bland foods; use saline gargles; and take analgesics, as needed.

Evaluation

Base your evaluation on the expected outcomes listed on the nursing care plan. To determine whether your patient has improved, ask yourself questions such as these:

- Does the patient use his leisure time meaningfully?
- Does he participate in a favorite hobby or chosen activity?

Sample nursing care plan: Infectious mononucleosis

Nursing diagnosis	**Expected outcomes**
Diversional activity deficit; related to fatigue and malaise	The patient will: • use leisure time meaningfully. • participate in a chosen activity, such as a hobby.
Nursing interventions	**Discharge planning**
• Schedule time for patient to pursue leisure activities. • Alternate treatments with rest periods to allow sufficient time for leisure activities. • Discuss patient's favorite topics while implementing procedures. • Collaborate with patient and family to develop ways to carry out desired activities.	• Review treatment plan with patient and family. • Help patient develop a schedule of diversional activities to participate in at home. • Explain to patient and family the importance of resting after activities. • To help prevent a relapse, advise patient not to tire himself.

Lymphocyte Disorders

The answers to these questions will help you evaluate your patient's status and the effectiveness of his care. Keep in mind that these questions stem from the sample care plan on page 132. Your questions may differ.

Acquired immune deficiency syndrome

A defect in cell-mediated (T cell) immunity that increases susceptibility to various opportunistic infections and unusual cancers characterizes acquired immune deficiency syndrome (AIDS). The immune defect results from infection with human immunodeficiency virus (HIV). Also known as lymphadenopathy-associated virus (LAV), human T cell lymphotropic virus type III (HTLV-III), and AIDS-related virus (ARV), this retrovirus contains ribonucleic acid (RNA) rather than deoxyribonucleic acid (DNA) as its genetic material. Present in an infected person's blood, semen, and other body fluids, HIV may spread during sex, from transfusion of contaminated blood or blood products, or from sharing an infected needle. The virus can also spread transplacentally, from an infected woman to her unborn child.

The incubation period for AIDS seems to last 2 to 7 years, possibly even longer. However, an infected person usually develops antibodies to the virus in 6 weeks to 6 months. A child infected in utero may show signs of AIDS when he's 2 months old. (See *Assessing for AIDS in a child*, page 136.)

The Centers for Disease Control (CDC) defines AIDS for surveillance purposes as the presence of an illness, such as an opportunistic infection or Kaposi's sarcoma (KS), that indicates defective cell-mediated immunity in a person with no known cause of immunosuppression other than HIV infection. The CDC recently broadened its definition of AIDS victims to include:

- presumptive cases, involving patients with signs of an AIDS-indicative disease but no known cause of immunosuppression, who haven't undergone HIV laboratory testing (or in whom results were inconclusive)—provided the AIDS-indicative disease has been diagnosed definitively
- patients with certain progressive, life-threatening, or disabling conditions (such as encephalopathy or wasting syndrome) that were not included under the old definition. Some patients with AIDS-related complex (ARC) fall into this category. ARC patients test positive for the HIV antibody but don't succumb to the opportunistic infections or cancers typical of AIDS. However, some do have wasting syndrome—chronic diarrhea and loss of more than 10% of body weight. Many ARC patients eventually develop full-blown AIDS.

Most American AIDS victims fall into one or more of these groups:

- homosexual or bisexual men
- I.V. drug users
- hemophiliacs and others who've received blood transfusions
- heterosexual partners of infected persons
- children born to infected women.

HIV usually infects the helper T lymphocyte (T_4 cell) but can also directly infect other cells, including B cells, macrophages, and cen-

Continued on page 134

Lymphocyte Disorders

How human immunodeficiency virus proliferates

After binding to a receptor on a T cell's surface, human immunodeficiency virus (HIV) penetrates the cell, transcribes its viral RNA into DNA, and becomes incorporated into the host cell genome. When antigenic stimulation activates the cell, the virus is expressed and eventually kills the cell. Viral particles released from the dead cell can then invade other T cells.

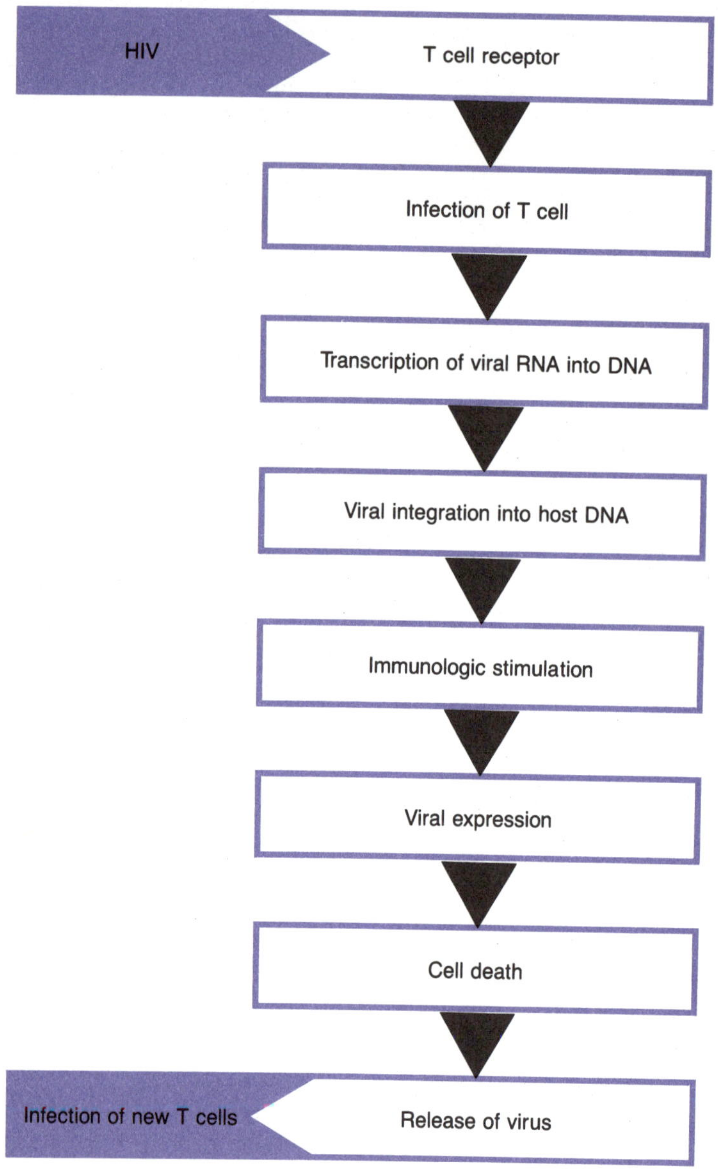

Acquired immune deficiency syndrome—*continued*

tral nervous system cells. Once inside a T_4 cell, the virus replicates with the help of a viral enzyme known as reverse transcriptase, then integrates into the cell's DNA. The abnormal T_4 cell that results makes copies of the virus, which then infect other cells. (See *How human immunodeficiency virus proliferates.*) Eventually, the number of normal T_4 cells drops so low that the immune system can no longer defend against the tumors and intracellular organisms (viruses, fungi, parasites, and mycobacteria) that T_4 cells usually attack. The immune system also can't carry out activities that rely

Lymphocyte Disorders

Common clinical syndromes accompanying AIDS

Gastrointestinal
- Cytomegalovirus (CMV)
- Cryptosporidiosis
- *Giardia lamblia* infection
- *Candida albicans* esophagitis/stomatitis
- Kaposi's sarcoma
- *Mycobacterium avium intracellulare*
- Human immunodeficiency virus (HIV) wasting syndrome

Neurologic
- *Toxoplasma gondii* encephalitis
- *Cryptococcus neoformans* meningitis
- CMV encephalitis
- HIV encephalopathy

Respiratory
- *Pneumocystis carinii* pneumonia
- CMV pneumonitis
- Pulmonary Kaposi's sarcoma
- *Mycobacterium avium intracellulare*
- *Mycobacterium tuberculosis*

Skin
- Kaposi's sarcoma lesions
- Herpes simplex virus abscesses
- Varicella zoster infection
- HIV infection

on T_4 cells for stimulation—natural killer cell function, macrophage function, and B cell response to new antigens.

AIDS complications can result from opportunistic and multiple infections, cancer, and drug toxicity. Complications most frequently involve the respiratory, GI, integumentary, and neurologic systems. Neurologic complications can result from direct infection of nervous system cells with HIV.

Common opportunistic infections include:
- *Pneumocystis carinii* pneumonia, causing shortness of breath, chest tightness or discomfort, cough, and fever
- *Candida albicans* stomatitis or esophagitis, causing white patchy spots, altered taste, difficulty swallowing, and retrosternal burning or pain
- *Toxoplasma gondii* encephalitis, causing headaches, confusion, subtle CNS changes, and seizures
- cryptosporidiosis, cytomegalovirus (CMV) infection, or parasitic infestation, causing severe diarrhea and abdominal discomfort.

A child with AIDS may develop interstitial pneumonitis and enlarged parotid glands as well as any of the opportunistic infections listed above.

With treatment, the AIDS patient may have alternating periods of illness and remission, lasting about 8 months to 2 years. During remission, he may feel healthy. Most AIDS patients eventually die of respiratory failure caused by CMV pneumonitis, *Pneumocystis carinii* pneumonia, or pulmonary KS.

Assessment

If you suspect your patient has AIDS, ask him whether he's recently experienced fever, night sweats, fatigue, weight loss, diarrhea, or abdominal discomfort. Also note any complaints of dyspnea; chest

Continued on page 136

Kaposi's sarcoma

This vascular tumor was rare in the U.S. and Europe until the outbreak of AIDS. It formerly affected elderly Jewish and Italian men, young black Africans, and patients with depressed immune function, commonly producing purple and brown plaques or nodules on the lower legs. The Kaposi's sarcoma associated with AIDS, although histologically identical to the rarer form, progresses more rapidly and typically involves many body sites, including the oral cavity, hard palate, gastrointestinal tract, lymph nodes, and lungs.

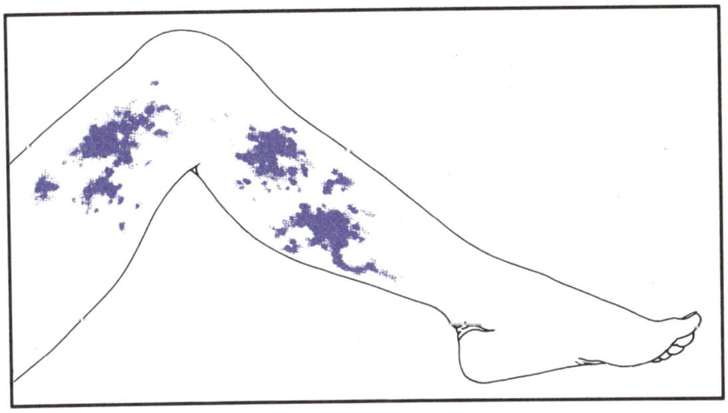

Lymphocyte Disorders

Assessing for AIDS in a child

A child infected with human immunodeficiency virus (HIV) during gestation typically begins to show signs and symptoms between age 2 and 4 months. Findings include fever, rashes, lymphadenopathy, chronic or recurrent diarrhea, liver and spleen enlargement, failure to thrive, microcephaly, and neurologic impairment. Craniofacial abnormalities, as shown in the illustration, may provide the first clue to infection. From age 4 months on, an infected child may test positive for HIV antibody (a younger child's immature immune system rules out diagnosis by this test).

Common clinical syndromes in pediatric AIDS patients include desquamative or lymphoid interstitial pneumonitis and fungal and bacterial infections. About 80% of these children develop *Pneumocystis carinii* pneumonia. Kaposi's sarcoma, common in adults with AIDS, rarely occurs in children.

In utero transmission of AIDS may cause the craniofacial abnormalities shown here.

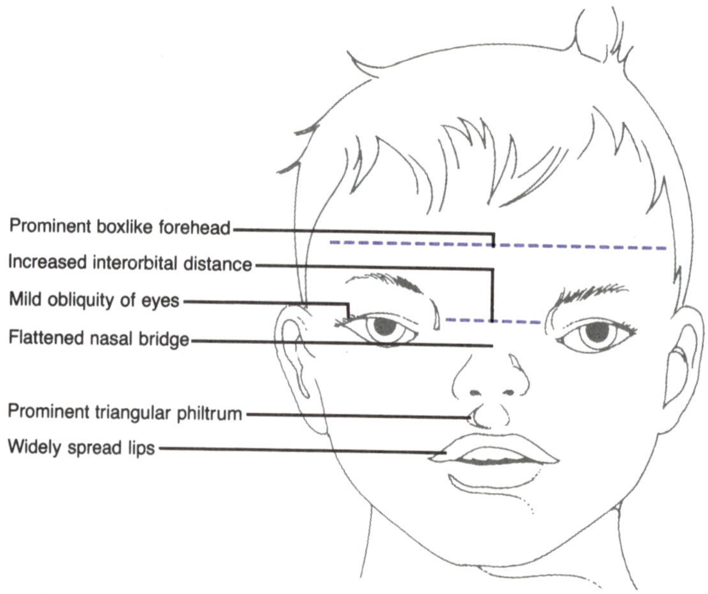

Acquired immune deficiency syndrome—*continued*

tightness or discomfort; cough; taste alteration; dysphagia; retrosternal burning or pain; or headaches, confusion, seizures, or other CNS symptoms.

Physical examination may reveal such abnormalities as hairy leukoplakia (lacy white patches on the oral mucosa); palpable purplish skin lesions (indicating Kaposi's sarcoma); and lymphadenopathy in neck, axillary, and groin nodes.

Diagnostic tests. Diagnosis rests on the patient's signs and symptoms and a positive test for HIV antibody. The test, enzyme-linked immunosorbent assay (ELISA), is always repeated when positive. To confirm ELISA results, the doctor will order the western blot analysis, a more specific antibody test. Blood banks now use ELISA to screen blood and blood products for AIDS contamination. However, an experimental test detects HIV infection sooner than the ELISA and western blot analysis. (See *New HIV antigen test.)*

Lymphocyte Disorders

New HIV antigen test

An experimental test can detect acquired immune deficiency syndrome (AIDS) infection earlier than other tests, speeding diagnosis, helping to monitor therapeutic effectiveness, and improving the safety of donated blood. Unlike the ELISA and western blot assays, the new test detects antigen from human immunodeficiency virus (HIV) rather than antibodies in blood samples. Antigen can appear in the blood a few days after HIV infection, while antibodies may not appear for 6 weeks to 6 months (or even longer). If an infected person donates blood before antibodies appear, his blood will test negative with the ELISA and western blot tests.

Researchers have used the antigen test to diagnose acute HIV infection, a flu-like condition that develops a few days to a few weeks after HIV exposure and lasts up to 10 days. Symptoms include sore throat, rash, and low-grade fever. All AIDS patients diagnosed by the antigen test later tested positive for HIV antibody.

A positive antibody test means that the patient has been infected with HIV. Although he may not have AIDS, he can transmit the virus through blood and sexual contact.

HIV can also be cultured from infected cells. Although it's too slow and difficult to be used for routine diagnosis, HIV culturing helps evaluate the effectiveness of experimental drugs.

Other diagnostic tests for AIDS include:
- a complete blood count with differential to check for lymphocytopenia
- an immune profile
- skin testing with common antigens to evaluate cell-mediated immunity.

Other tests may be necessary to diagnose opportunistic infections or AIDS-related cancers. For instance, biopsies diagnose KS lesions; bronchial washings or transbronchial biopsy taken during bronchoscopy help diagnose *Pneumocystis carinii* pneumonia; cultures help diagnose *Candida albicans* and herpes simplex.

Planning

Focus your nursing care on preventing or controlling the potentially fatal opportunistic infections that pose a threat to the AIDS patient. Care goals include assisting with measures to treat infection, maintaining patient comfort, helping the patient cope with his diagnosis, and teaching him about infection control and follow-up care.

Nursing diagnoses. Before determining your nursing care plan, develop the nursing diagnosis by identifying the patient's actual or potential problem, then relating it to its cause. Possible nursing diagnoses for a patient with AIDS include:
- infection, potential for; related to debilitation and malnutrition
- nutrition, alteration in (less than body requirements); related to anorexia, oral pain, dysphagia, and increased metabolism
- activity intolerance; related to fatigue, malaise, and tissue hypoxia
- oral mucous membrane, alteration in; related to stomatitis
- comfort, alteration in (chills and excessive diaphoresis); related to fever
- self-care deficit (total); related to activity intolerance
- anxiety; related to diagnosis and its implications
- coping, ineffective individual; related to depression associated with diagnosis, poor prognosis, and inadequate support system
- sleep pattern disturbance; related to anxiety and discomfort
- sexual dysfunction (decreased libido); related to fatigue, weakness, anxiety, depression and/or fear
- knowledge deficit; related to infection control measures
- grieving, anticipatory; related to potential premature death.

The sample nursing care plan on page 138 shows expected outcomes, nursing interventions, and discharge planning for one nursing diagnosis listed above. However, you'll want to tailor each care plan to fit your patient's needs.

Intervention

Although AIDS remains incurable, the patient can be treated for opportunistic infections and cancers. For some patients, the doctor

Continued on page 138

Lymphocyte Disorders

Sample nursing care plan: Acquired immune deficiency syndrome (AIDS)

Nursing diagnosis	Expected outcomes
Knowledge deficit; related to infection control measures	The patient will: • describe signs and symptoms of opportunistic infections. • state ways to reduce the risk of opportunistic infections.
Nursing interventions	**Discharge planning**
• Teach patient signs and symptoms of opportunistic infections, such as fever; chills; persistent headache; perianal itching and/or pain; and frequency, urgency, or burning on urination. • Advise patient how to reduce the risk of contracting an opportunistic infection, such as by: regularly cleaning kitchen and bathroom surfaces (especially shower floor) with a disinfectant to prevent fungal growth using gloves when cleaning birdcages and cat litter boxes to avoid *psittacosis* and *toxoplasmosis* exposure keeping the home well-ventilated to reduce exposure to airborne diseases avoiding contact with persons who have an infection (particularly viral) or who have recently been vaccinated balancing rest with activity staying alert for and promptly reporting signs and symptoms of infection informing all health care providers of AIDS diagnosis so they won't prescribe immunosuppressant drugs, such as corticosteroids eating a healthful diet and drinking at least 10 glasses (approximately 2,400 ml) of liquid daily.	• Provide patient, partner, and family with information about resources to help them cope with AIDS (including AIDS hotlines, Public Health Service, Centers for Disease Control, and National Gay Task Force). If necessary, refer them for counseling. • Consult with community health nurse to provide follow-up care at home, as indicated. • Review treatment and teaching plans with patient, partner, and family. Answer questions they might have. • Explain the actions and adverse effects of all medications. Reinforce the importance of compliance with the treatment regimen. • Remind patient to keep scheduled follow-up medical appointments.

Acquired immune deficiency syndrome—*continued*

may order zidovudine (Retrovir), formerly called AZT, a drug that seems to block HIV replication. Available in oral form, Retrovir causes fewer adverse effects than many other drugs under study. Retrovir's adverse effects include headache, rash, anemia, leukopenia, and granulocytopenia. (In one study, about 25% of patients receiving Retrovir needed blood transfusions after 4 to 8 weeks of therapy.) Scientists are testing other drugs, including ampligen, suramin, ribavirin, alpha-interferon, and HPA-23. (See *Anti-AIDS drugs: An update.)*

Aside from such drugs, AIDS treatment remains supportive, attempting to cure or control complications as they develop. For example, the doctor may order single-agent or combination chemotherapy to treat KS, although combination chemotherapy's usually reserved for life-threatening KS because its side effects can be lethal. The most common agents, vinblastine (Velban) and etoposide (VePesid), suppress bone marrow function, which may further impair immune function. Radiation has been successful for palliative or cosmetic purposes, but hasn't proved useful as a systemic approach. Alpha-interferon has induced partial or complete KS remission in about 30% of patients studied. This therapy seems to

Lymphocyte Disorders

Anti-AIDS drugs: An update

A new family of drugs designed to inhibit the human immunodeficiency virus (HIV) from reproducing may prove effective against AIDS. One of these drugs, zidovudine (Retrovir), formerly known as AZT, won approval from the Food and Drug Administration in 1986.

Zidovudine appears to work by inhibiting reverse transcriptase, an enzyme essential for HIV proliferation. HIV proliferates by imposing reverse transcriptase over the host cell's genetic code, transforming it into a virus producer. Zidovudine closely resembles this enzyme, confusing the virus into using the drug rather than the necessary enzyme. As a result, the virus loses its reproductive ability, which may help stabilize the patient's condition and allow his immune system to regenerate.

Though it does cause considerable adverse side effects, oral zidovudine causes fewer adverse effects than many other drugs under study.

Drugs currently undergoing clinical trials in AIDS patients include ampligen, suramin, ribavirin, alpha-interferon, and the French drug HPA-23.

Ampligen. Classified as a biological response modifier, ampligen has a dual effect. It:
- inhibits HIV by unblocking the activity of RNAse L, a virus-destroying enzyme whose activity HIV blocks
- stimulates the immune system.

The drug has no apparent adverse effects.

In recent studies, most patients with AIDS-related complex (ARC) and lymphadenopathy syndrome (LAS)—precursors of AIDS—improved markedly with ampligen treatment; patients with full-blown AIDS improved less dramatically. Based on these results, researchers believe that ampligen alone may provide effective treatment for patients with early stage AIDS. For advanced disease, the drug may become the foundation of combination regimens.

Because it's synergistic with zidovudine and alpha-interferon, ampligen may increase the effectiveness of these drugs while reducing their toxicity when given concomitantly.

work best for patients with the strongest immune profiles. Some doctors recommend no therapy for KS unless it's making the patient ill.

Many agents that fight opportunistic infections cause serious adverse effects in AIDS patients. What's more, when therapy stops, many infections recur. For *Pneumocystis carinii,* for example, the doctor usually prescribes oral or I.V. co-trimoxazole (Bactrim, Septra). Its common adverse effects include hypersensitivity, rash, and leukopenia. If treatment fails or toxicity occurs, the doctor may order I.M. or I.V. pentamidine (Pentam 300), which can damage the kidneys or liver and cause hyperglycemia or hypoglycemia and hypotension.

For a patient with *Toxoplasma gondii* encephalitis, the doctor will probably order a combination of pyrimethamine (Daraprim) and sulfadiazine (Microsulfan). Adverse effects include hypersensitivity reactions and bone marrow suppression. The patient will probably require long-term therapy.

Candida albicans can be treated with nystatin or clotrimazole; severe cases may warrant ketoconazole or amphotericin B. Treatment for *Cryptococcus neoformans* meningitis involves I.V. amphotericin B, usually in combination with flucytosine. Amphotericin B is highly toxic, especially to the kidneys. Herpes simplex lesions usually respond to I.V. or P.O. acyclovir; the patient may need the drug chronically.

Currently, no standard treatment's available for *Cryptosporidium, Mycobacterium avium intracellulare,* or CMV infection. However, a new agent known as DHPG shows promise in treating CMV infections.

Nursing intervention. The AIDS patient requires comprehensive, careful, and continuous assessment. Watch for signs and symptoms of common clinical syndromes and complications, which can be subtle. Early detection and intervention can markedly influence treatment outcome. Include these nursing measures in your care:
- Monitor the patient's respiratory status. If he has respiratory problems, position him properly, provide oxygen, and pace his activities to prevent overexertion. As ordered, give antimicrobials promptly according to the dosage schedule.
- Regularly assess the patient's neurologic and mental status. If he has a CNS infection, he may need reality orientation and safety precautions. As ordered and needed, take seizure precautions and administer anticonvulsants.
- Closely monitor the patient's nutritional and electrolyte status, especially if he has diarrhea. He may need supplemental, high-calorie feedings or I.V. hyperalimentation. Antidiarrheals, such as diphenoxylate (Lomotil) or tincture of opium, may help. Be sure to provide meticulous mouth care, using rinses with normal saline solution plus hydrogen peroxide or sodium bicarbonate to maintain hygiene and comfort.
- Monitor KS or herpes simplex lesions and encourage or provide good skin care. Herpes lesions, usually painful, may necessitate analgesic drug treatment and a careful regimen for wound healing.

Continued on page 140

Lymphocyte Disorders

Caring for AIDS patients: Infection control guidelines

When caring for a hospitalized AIDS patient, impose blood and body fluid precautions for infection control, as described here:

- Wash hands before and after contact with the patient or with any soiled items.
- Wear gloves to avoid contact with blood or body fluids, or with objects and materials soiled with them.
- Wear a gown if a chance exists that your clothing will be soiled with the patient's blood or body fluids.
- Wear a mask only if a possibility exists that blood or other secretions will splash in your face, for example, when suctioning a patient or while assisting with an endoscopy.
- Dispose of needles in an accessible, impervious container as soon as possible after use. Needles should not be bent, cut, or resheathed.
- Label laboratory specimens "Blood and Body Fluid Precautions" and place in a plastic bag for transport.
- Label and bag linen according to hospital policy for infection control precautions.
- Clean blood spills with a 1:10 solution of sodium hypochlorite 5.25% (household bleach).
- Visitors don't need to take precautions unless they might come into contact with the patient's blood or body fluids.

Keep in mind that some hospitals have adopted universal precautions for nurses to follow when contacting any patient's secretions. Check with your employer about specific policies and precautions.

Acquired immune deficiency syndrome—*continued*

- Encourage healthy behaviors, such as good nutrition, rest, exercise as tolerated, good hygiene, and infection prevention. Teach your patient the signs and symptoms of infection and what to do if these appear.
- Explain how to avoid transmitting AIDS to others. Provide the patient with information about safe sex practices. Instruct him not to donate blood, organs, or semen and not to share razors, toothbrushes, or other items that might be contaminated with blood. Urge a woman to avoid pregnancy. Advise the patient to inform doctors, dentists, and sexual partners of the diagnosis.
- Be prepared to deal with the patient's psychosocial concerns. Besides the prognosis of a terminal illness and the isolation of social disapproval, the AIDS patient must face rapid and severe body changes that can crush self-esteem. Some patients lose their jobs, financial security, and health insurance. Many lose family support because of geographic distance, emotional separation, or family members' fears for their own health. Friends and family may simply not know what to do. You can help by offering support to the patient, helping him maintain hope (while remaining realistic about his prognosis), teaching him what he needs to know to cope with his disease, and referring him and the people close to him for appropriate counseling.

Evaluation

Base your evaluation on the expected outcomes listed on the nursing care plan. To determine whether your patient has improved, ask youself these questions:

- Can the patient describe signs and symptoms of infection?
- Can he explain how to decrease the risk of opportunistic infection?

The answers to these questions will help you evaluate your patient's status and the effectiveness of your care. Keep in mind that these questions stem from the sample nursing care plan on page 138. Your questions may differ.

Note: Ongoing AIDS research continues to provide new and important information on this deadly disease. In the NURSEREVIEW section "Immune Problems," you'll find additional information on AIDS research and patient care.

Plasma Cell, Monocyte, and Macrophage Disorders: Myeloma and Other Problems

Joan E. Mason, who wrote this chapter, is a Nurse Consultant and Clinical Editor at Springhouse Corporation. Ms. Mason formerly held positions as Nursing Instructor at Philadelphia General Hospital School of Nursing and as Staff Education Director at Roxborough Memorial Hospital, Philadelphia. She received her BS in Nursing Education and her master's degree in Health Education from Temple University, Philadelphia.

In this chapter, we'll discuss major plasma cell disorders—plasma cell myeloma, Waldenström's macroglobulinemia, and heavy-chain diseases—as well as a few monocyte and macrophage problems. Before reading about these disorders, first review some basics about plasma cells, monocytes, and macrophages.

Plasma cell development, structure, and function. Plasma cells, which exist in lymphatic and connective tissue throughout the body, can originate in two ways. Most develop from lymphocytes; after antigenic stimulation, some B lymphocytes differentiate into plasma cells. This conversion's highly specific, triggered only by antigens that chemically and physically match the B cell's antibodies.

Some plasma cells develop from a maturation pathway starting with a stem cell that matures into a plasmablast, then a proplasmacyte, and, finally, a plasma cell, or plasmacyte.

The mature plasma cell is round or oval and contains a cartwheel nucleus: a structure with deeply staining chromatin material arranged in a spokelike pattern.

With some diseases, plasma cells may become abnormal in size or shape (as in myeloma) and may contain abnormal inclusions (for example, hemosiderin inclusions in hemochromatosis and hemosiderosis).

Because they're the main source of immunoglobulins (antibodies), plasma cells play an important role in immune functions.

Immunoglobulins. These plasma cell products fall into five classes based on structure and function: IgG, IgM, IgA, IgD, and IgE. (See *Immunoglobulins: Variations on a Y-shaped monomer,* page 142.) IgG, IgM, and IgA have identifiable subclasses.

IgG. The major immunoglobulin in the blood, IgG constitutes about 75% of the serum immunoglobulin fraction. It's also found in extravascular fluids: lymph, cerebrospinal fluid, synovial fluid, and peritoneal fluid. The IgG molecule's the smallest of the immunoglobulins; its bivalent Y-shaped monomeric structure allows only two antigen-binding sites, one on each arm of the Y.

IgG is the second immunoglobulin (after IgM) to respond to an antigen in a primary immune response, but it's the major immunoglobulin to respond after reexposure to the antigen (secondary, anamnestic antibody response). After IgG combines with an antigen, the immunoglobulin's Fc portion (stem of the IgG monomer) can bind to the first component of the classical complement pathway; this activates the complement cascade, by which the humoral immune response takes place.

IgM. Found mainly in the blood, IgM constitutes about 10% of the serum immunoglobulin fraction. The largest immunoglobulin, IgM has a structure incorporating five Y-shaped monomeric units (arranged radially in a star-shaped molecule known as a pentamer) with a small polypeptide chain (J chain). Therefore, each IgM molecule contains 10 potential antigen-binding sites. However, apparently not all sites bind with equal efficiency, and up to half may not bind at all.

Continued on page 142

Normal plasma cell

A mature plasma cell contains an eccentrically placed nucleus and a deeply staining chromatin mass, as shown in this illustrated electron micrograph.

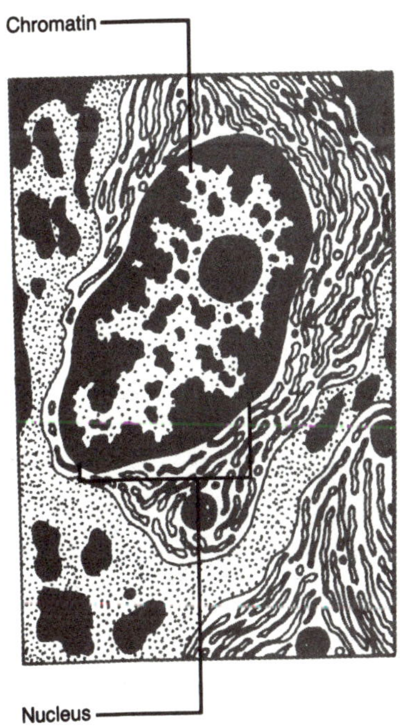

Plasma Cell and Other Disorders

Immunoglobulins: Variations on a Y-shaped monomer

Immunoglobulins, large protein molecules, consist of four polypeptide chains: two long, *heavy* (H) chains and two short, *light* (L) chains. Each L chain is linked to an H chain, and the two H chains are linked to each other by disulfide bonds.

The basic structure (monomeric unit) of an immunoglobulin is Y-shaped. The two arms of the Y contain the *antigen-binding fragment* (Fab). Thus, immunoglobulin monomers are bivalent, having two antigen-binding sites, one at the end of each arm.

The outer portion of the Fab region, where variable sequences of polypeptide chains reside, defines the character of the antigen-binding site and is known as the *variable* (V) region. The inner Fab region is known as the *constant* (C) region because of the constancy of the amino acid sequence.

The stem of the Y is known as the *crystallizable fragment* (Fc). This area, part of the C region, contains the disulfide bonds that link the H chains. The Fc region participates in effector functions of immunoglobulins, such as activation of complement, and provides a binding site for Fc receptors on phagocytic cells. The major structural differences among IgG, IgM, IgA, IgE, and IgD are in the H chains, which are specific for each class.

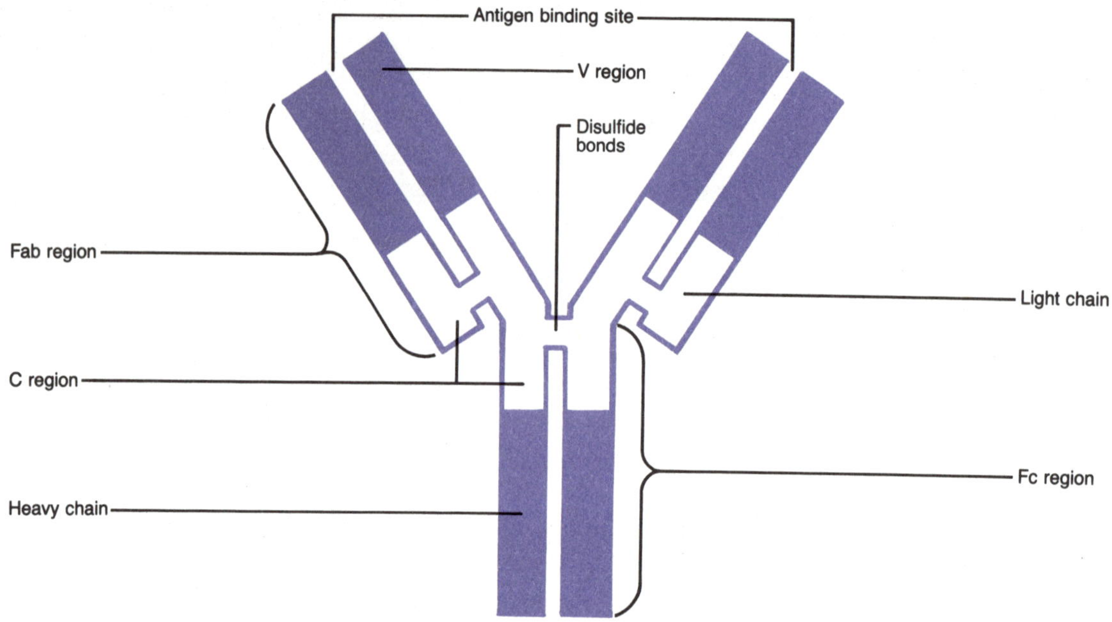

Continued

IgM is the first immunoglobulin to respond to an antigen and the major antibody involved in the primary immune response. It functions like IgG but activates the complement system more effectively, triggering the complement cascade by binding with viral and bacterial antigens.

IgA. This immunoglobulin exists in two types: serum IgA and secretory IgA. Serum IgA accounts for about 10% to 15% of the serum immunoglobulin fraction and usually consists of one Y-shaped monomeric unit. Secretory IgA, the predominant form, consists of two IgA molecules and a J chain bound to a secretory component by disulfide bonds. It's concentrated in the exocrine secretions, such as colostrum, milk, tears, sweat, and saliva, and in other respiratory, gastrointestinal, and urogenital secretions. At these potential antigen entry sites, it provides specific antibody protection against pathogens.

IgD. This immunoglobulin makes up less than 1% of the serum immunoglobulin fraction. Found on the surface of B cells, it may play a role in their differentiation.

Plasma Cell and Other Disorders

IgE. This immunoglobulin's normally present in only trace amounts. Elevated levels usually appear in allergic disorders and certain parasitic infections. Most IgE-producing cells exist in the respiratory and intestinal mucosa. IgE functions mainly in allergic reactions; its Fc region binds with high affinity to mast cells and basophils, leaving its Fab region (the antigen-binding fragment of the Y arm) free to bind with an allergen (an antigen that can produce an allergic reaction). When two or more IgE molecules bind to an allergen, mast cells or basophils release histamine, kinins, serotonin, leukotrienes, and neutrophil chemotactic factor. These chemical mediators, in turn, produce the characteristic wheal-and-flare allergic skin reaction, allergic (extrinsic) asthma, and allergic seasonal rhinitis (hay fever).

Monocyte and macrophage development, structure, and function. Monocytes and macrophages are agranulocytes formed in the bone marrow. Monocytes are the largest white blood cells (WBCs), ranging up to about 20 microns in diameter. They circulate from the blood to the tissues, concentrating in areas of infection. After several hours in tissue spaces, they swell, maturing into macrophages—powerful phagocytes that can engulf up to 100 bacteria. Macrophages are especially effective in eliminating large particles of cell debris and worn-out red blood cells (RBCs). With chronic inflammation, serum monocytes may increase sharply, accounting for 30% to 50% of all WBCs. Immature monocytes that become fixed in the tissue are called tissue macrophages, or histiocytes. These cells establish themselves in lymph nodes, pulmonary alveoli, the spleen, the bone marrow, and the hepatic sinuses (where they're known as Kupffer's cells).

Plasma cell myeloma

Also known as multiple myeloma, plasma cell myeloma (PCM) is the most common plasma cell cancer. Plasma cells in the bone marrow proliferate uncontrollably and infiltrate bone to produce osteolytic lesions throughout the skeleton. Common tumor (plasmacytoma) sites include the skull, jaw, scapulae, sternum, clavicles, vertebrae, pelvis, and ribs. Rarely, a tumor may originate in extraskeletal sites (nasopharynx, paranasal sinuses, larynx, thorax, paravertebral or epidural tissues, lymph nodes, or GI tract). A plasmacytoma that first appears solitary usually becomes generalized. In its late stages, the disease infiltrates the liver, spleen, lymph nodes, lungs, adrenal glands, kidneys, skin, and GI tract.

For a period ranging from months to years, the plasmacytoma grows from a few millimeters to several centimeters in diameter. Usually multiple, these pink or reddish tumors are firm and fleshy. They may erode adjacent bone and compress the spinal cord or nerve roots emanating from the spinal canal.

Abnormal plasma cell growth can produce such pathophysiologic changes as osteolysis, hematopoietic suppression (from malignant cell infiltration of the marrow, which inhibits RBC production), hypogammaglobulinemia (which increases the infection risk), paraproteinemia, and renal disease. Hypercalcemia also can occur from reduced renal calcium excretion and inactivity, both of which pro-

Continued on page 144

Plasma Cell and Other Disorders

Osteolytic lesions

This section of an osteolytic lesion in a patient with plasma cell myeloma shows plasma cells as the darkly stained cells not contacting bone; the large, multinucleated cells are osteoclasts.

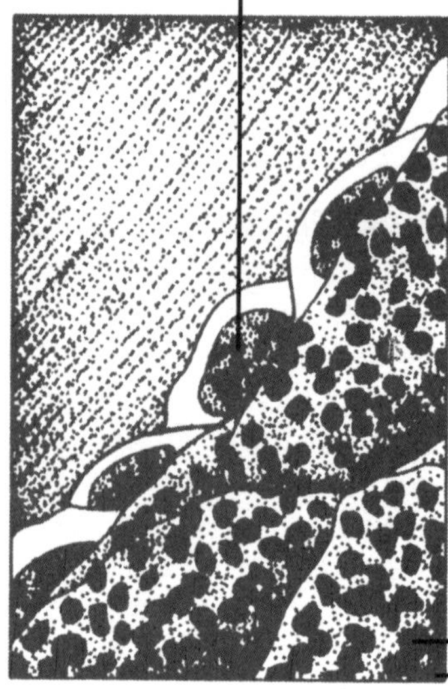

This illustration of an X-ray shows an osteolytic lesion typical of plasma cell myeloma.

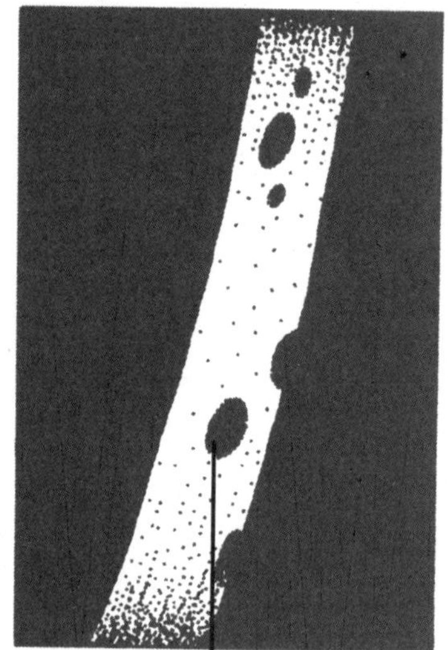

Plasma cell myeloma—*continued*

mote calcium mobilization from the skeleton. The patient commonly experiences hypercalcemia within 1 month after he's bedridden with painful skeletal lesions. Inactivity may trigger a cycle of hypercalciuria, which leads to osmotic diuresis and impaired renal tubular reabsorption, leading to dehydration. This causes reduced renal output, resulting in hypercalcemia and azotemia, producing nausea, vomiting, and further dehydration.

PCM commonly leads to impaired marrow function, to a degree reflecting the marrow's plasma cell level. The mechanism causing marrow dysfunction remains unknown. The hallmark of PCM is the production of an abnormal monoclonal immunoglobulin, indicated by the presence of Bence Jones protein in the urine. This protein constitutes the light chain component of myeloma globulin. Filtered by the glomeruli, it's then reabsorbed and metabolized. Bence Jones protein spills into the urine when it exceeds the tubules' capacity to reabsorb it. Renal tubules degenerate from this effort to reabsorb excessive amounts of protein, thus severely damaging the kidneys. Hyperuricosuria, hypercalciuria, and nephrocalcinosis may worsen renal function. Hyperuricemia results from increased cellular turnover, causing uric acid crystallization and subsequent renal tubule obstruction, adding to renal failure. Dehydration poses the greatest threat to a severely ill patient. Infection and, in late disease stages, severe plasma cell infiltration of the kidney may occur, further impairing renal function.

PCM accounts for about 10% of all hematologic cancers and 1% of all cancers. More common in men, it affects twice as many blacks as whites. The disease has a poor prognosis because diagnosis

Plasma Cell and Other Disorders

commonly comes after the disease has infiltrated various bones. By then, skeletal destruction's widespread. Untreated, PCM leads to vertebral collapse. About half of PCM patients die within 3 months of diagnosis, 90% within 2 years. However, early diagnosis and treatment can prolong the lives of some patients by 3 to 5 years. Death usually follows complications, such as hypercalcemia, infection, renal failure, neurologic impairment, or hyperviscosity syndrome.

Neurologic impairment presents as spinal cord compression, resulting in paraplegia, or as a direct involvement of nerve tissue, causing neuropathies and cranial nerve abnormalities (hearing loss).

Hyperviscosity syndrome stems from production of abnormal immunoglobulins. It may cause fatigue; weakness; skin, mucosal, and GI bleeding; visual disturbances; headache; and other neurologic problems.

Assessment

Ask yourself these questions when taking your patient's history and performing the physical examination:

- Does the patient complain of *bone pain?* The most common PCM symptom, bone pain stems from diffuse or localized osteolytic areas located near focal points of abnormal plasma cell growth. Lower back or rib pain exacerbated by movement develops gradually or fluctuates in intensity for weeks or months, then becomes disabling. Sudden severe pain usually signals vertebral collapse or spontaneous fracture through a diseased region of the pelvis, the clavicle, a long bone shaft, or a rib. The patient's height may decrease from vertebral collapse.
- Does the patient report *systemic symptoms?* These may include weakness, fatigue, pallor, palpitations, and dyspnea on exertion (partly from concurrent anemia). Thrombocytopenia may cause purpura, epistaxis, or excessive bleeding after injury. Immunoglobulin deficiencies and neutropenia may produce signs and symptoms of such infections as pneumonia, pyoderma, or pyelonephritis. Cryoglobulinemia may lead to cold sensitivity and urticaria. Edema may also occur.
- Does the patient have signs or symptoms of *hypercalcemia?* These may include anorexia, nausea, vomiting, constipation, dehydration, muscle flaccidity, pathologic fractures, and flank pain (associated with renal calculi). Eventually, drowsiness, confusion, and coma develop.
- Does the patient have signs or symptoms of *hyperviscosity* (as described earlier)?
- Does the patient have signs or symptoms of *infection,* such as fever, chills, night sweats, malaise, fatigue, coughing, and dyspnea? PCM, which increases susceptibility to infection, is sometimes diagnosed during an episode of pneumonia or infection of the upper respiratory tract, paranasal sinuses, throat, skin, or urinary passages.
- Does the patient have signs of *spinal cord or nerve root compression?* Radicular pain, a common early sign, is usually well localized to a dermatome and exacerbated by coughing, sneezing, or straining. Late findings include sensory and motor loss and paraplegia.

Continued on page 146

Plasma Cell and Other Disorders

Bence Jones protein

The hallmark of plasma cell myeloma, this protein (a light chain of gamma globulin) was named for Henry Bence Jones, an English doctor who in 1848 noticed that patients with a curious bone disease excreted a unique protein—unique in that it coagulated at 113° to 131° F. (45° to 55° C.), then redissolved when heated to boiling. Otto Kahler, an Austrian, demonstrated in 1889 that Bence Jones protein was related to myeloma. Bence Jones protein is not found in the urine of *all* patients with plasma cell myeloma, but it is almost never found in patients without this disease.

Plasma cell myeloma—*continued*

Diagnostic tests. The following studies help confirm PCM:

- *Blood tests.* Complete blood count reveals moderate to severe anemia. The differential may show 40% to 50% lymphocytes but seldom more than 3% plasma cells. Rouleaux formation (commonly the first clue) seen on differential smear stems from an elevated erythrocyte sedimentation rate. Serum calcium and phosphorus levels may rise above normal; hemoglobin level may drop below normal; platelet count usually decreases.
- *Urine studies.* These may show Bence Jones protein and hypercalciuria. Although absence of this protein doesn't rule out PCM, its presence almost invariably confirms it. Plasma cells may appear in urinary sediment.
- *Bone marrow aspiration.* This reveals an abnormal number of immature plasma cells.
- *Serum electrophoresis.* This shows an elevated globulin spike that's electrophoretically and immunologically abnormal.
- *X-rays.* During early stages, these may show only diffuse osteoporosis. Eventually, they show multiple, sharply circumscribed, osteolytic (punched-out) lesions, particularly on the skull, pelvis, and spine.
- *Excretory urography.* This test determines renal involvement. To avoid precipitation of Bence Jones protein, the doctor uses iothalamate or diatrizoate instead of the usual contrast medium. (*Note:* Although oral fluids are usually restricted before excretory urography, the patient with PCM should receive copious fluids, usually orally, but sometimes I.V.)
- *Immunologic tests.* These may reveal abnormal immunoglobulin levels.

Planning

Focus your nursing care on controlling pain and teaching your patient how to prevent complications.

Nursing diagnoses. Before determining your nursing care plan, develop the nursing diagnosis by identifying the patient's actual or potential problem, then relating it to its cause. Possible nursing diagnoses for a patient with PCM include the following:

- comfort, alteration in (pain); related to vertebral collapse or pathologic fracture
- mobility, impaired physical; related to bone fragility and pain
- activity intolerance; related to immobility associated with pain
- breathing patterns, ineffective; related to immobilization
- comfort, alteration in (sensitivity to cold); related to reduced circulation associated with hyperviscosity syndrome
- injury, potential for (spontaneous fractures or falls); related to weak, brittle bones
- infection, potential for; related to B cell dysfunction
- urinary elimination, alteration in; related to an increased serum calcium level.

The sample nursing care plan on the next page shows expected outcomes, nursing interventions, and discharge planning for one nursing diagnosis listed above. However, you'll want to tailor each care plan to fit your patient's needs.

Plasma Cell and Other Disorders

Sample nursing care plan: Plasma cell myeloma

Nursing diagnosis	Expected outcomes
Comfort, alteration in (pain); related to vertebral collapse or pathologic fracture	The patient will: • verbalize his pain. • identify factors that exacerbate or alleviate pain. • state when he feels pain relief.
Nursing interventions	**Discharge planning**
• Assess patient for pain. • Explain to patient why he has pain and how long it may last. • Implement behavioral measures, such as therapeutic touch, relaxation therapy, or guided imagery. • Perform comfort measures, such as repositioning, to promote relaxation. • Plan activities, such as crafts, reading, or television, to provide distraction. • Monitor and record effectiveness of administered pain medications. • Schedule treatments to allow uninterrupted rest periods.	• Consult with physical therapist and community health nurse to provide care at home. • Remind patient to alternate activity with rest. • Teach patient the actions, interactions, and adverse effects of pain medications he'll take home. • Instruct patient to take an analgesic before activities so that its peak effect occurs during the activity. • Review comfort measures that patient can use at home. • Schedule patient for follow-up medical appointments as necessary.

Intervention

Long-term treatment involves chemotherapy and adjuvant local radiation therapy to alleviate pain and reduce acute lesions. Other possible treatments include surgery, interferon, and various drugs and procedures to manage any special problems.

Chemotherapy. About half of PCM patients improve when given such alkylating agents as melphalan (Alkeran), cyclophosphamide (Cytoxan, Neosar), chlorambucil (Leukeran), and carmustine (BCNU [BiCNU]). Most alkylating agents are equally toxic to resting and proliferating cells. However, cyclophosphamide's much more toxic to proliferating marrow cells than to resting marrow cells. This drug's also more effective when given in intermittent doses rather than daily doses of comparable toxicity; this may stem partly from the drug's increasingly toxic effect on hematopoietic cells during daily administration, as injured cells are replaced by stem cells drawn into the cycle. Thus, large intermittent doses allow the marrow to recover.

Intermittent administration of melphalan and carmustine permits the doctor to see the patient every 4 to 6 weeks to obtain blood counts and serum and/or urinary monoclonal protein measurements. If the doctor orders small daily doses of an alkylating agent, the patient may need more frequent blood counts.

Prednisone therapy inhibits osteoclast activation and reduces bone resorption, thus relieving hypercalcemia. It also lowers the concentration of serum proteins, including monoclonal proteins, and may significantly raise the hematocrit level. Continued marrow plasmacytosis suggests that prednisone reduces monoclonal protein levels by inducing protein hypercatabolism rather than through a direct action on myeloma cells. Protein hypercatabolism produces a negative nitrogen balance and lowers the serum protein level. However, prednisone therapy alone can reduce tumor size and thus may have a direct antineoplastic action. (*Note:* Calcitonin [Calcimar]

Continued on page 148

Plasma Cell and Other Disorders

Plasma cell myeloma: Common therapies

For plasma cell growth suppression
- adrenocorticotropic hormone (ACTH)
- corticosteroids
- cyclophosphamide (Cytoxan)
- mechlorethamine (Mustargen)
- melphalan (Alkeran)
- radiation therapy

For bone remineralization
- activity (including physical therapy)
- anabolic steroids
- androgens
- calcium
- fluoride
- vitamin D

For stimulation of blood cell formation
- androgens

For pain relief
- bed rest
- orthopedic supports
- physical therapy
- analgesics

Plasma cell myeloma—*continued*

also helps treat hypercalcemia. The doctor may order this drug concomitantly with prednisone until the serum calcium level normalizes—usually within 1 to 5 days.)

Interferon. This experimental treatment has inhibited tumor cell proliferation and induced visible improvement in a few patients, achieving long-lasting remissions.

Radiation therapy. This provides palliative relief for patients with localized lesions, including large osteolytic long-bone lesions (which may lead to fracture), extraskeletal tumors, osteolytic vertebral lesions, and plasma cell tumors that compress the spinal cord or nerve roots.

The doctor may also order radiation therapy for a patient who has a solitary plasmacytoma. Unless the lesion's not truly solitary, radiation will eliminate urinary monoclonal proteins and restore a normal plasma cell level in bone marrow. (*Note:* Monoclonal proteins in serum or urine, or plasmacytosis following radiation therapy, indicates the need for chemotherapy.)

Surgery. The doctor may perform a laminectomy if a plasmacytoma causes acute spinal compression.

Managing special problems. If the patient becomes febrile, which suggests infection, the doctor will order cultures of blood, urine, sputum, skin lesions, or other potential infection sites. The most common infections include septicemia and those resulting from penicillin-resistant staphylococci and gram-negative organisms. Expect the doctor to begin antibiotic therapy before culture and antibiotic sensitivity results are available. For a serious infection, he'll probably start with antibiotic combinations that attack penicillin-resistant staphylococci and gram-negative organisms. Stay alert for indications of nephrotoxicity when caring for a patient who's receiving these drugs.

A patient with recurrent infection by sensitive organisms (for example, pneumococci) may benefit from prophylactic long-acting penicillin (penicillin G benzathine).

If the patient has hyperviscosity syndrome, plasmapheresis may be effective. This procedure helps normalize plasma volume and brings the relative serum viscosity below four times that of water by removing plasma containing monoclonal proteins, thus temporarily relieving symptoms of bleeding or congestive heart failure (CHF). Plasmapheresis also helps correct cryoglobulinemia.

The doctor may order androgen therapy (for example, fluoxymesterone [Android-F]) for a patient with persistent anemia caused by marrow failure (rather than by bleeding, folic acid or vitamin B_{12} deficiency, or chemotherapy). Androgens usually elevate the hemoglobin level.

Hyperuricemia—a common finding with PCM—may stem from renal insufficiency. Thus, therapy, usually involving daily allopurinol (Lopurin, Zyloprim) doses, aims to improve renal function by preventing development of renal calculi or nephropathy.

Plasma Cell and Other Disorders

When a patient experiences acute renal failure from excessive light-chain excretion, treatment aims to reduce the renal light-chain load. Plasmapheresis proves about 10 times more effective than peritoneal dialysis in light-chain removal. The doctor will also start chemotherapy at once. Improved renal function persists as long as myeloma cell growth remains under control.

To manage bone demineralization and osteolytic skeletal lesions (possibly resulting in disabling bone pain and fractures), the doctor will order treatment aimed at recalcifying bone, such as sodium fluoride or calcium lactate, or he may order both drugs given concomitantly with vitamin D to ensure proper bone mineralization. Experts recommend daily doses of 50 mg of sodium fluoride and at least 900 mg of calcium, with twice-weekly doses of 50,000 units of vitamin D. Androgens help achieve maximal bone strengthening. Some patients may require orthopedic braces for support.

Nursing intervention. Besides administering the drugs and other treatments discussed above, as ordered, also take these measures when caring for a patient with PCM:

- Encourage intake of 3,000 to 4,000 ml of fluids daily (particularly before excretory urography). Monitor intake and output (daily output shouldn't fall below 1,500 ml).
- Advise the patient to walk (immobilization promotes bone demineralization and susceptibility to pneumonia). Give analgesics, as ordered, for pain. Assign someone to walk with him or make sure he uses a walker or other supportive aid to prevent falls. If the patient's fearful (because of his increased risk for pathologic fractures), reassure him and let him proceed at his own pace.
- Prevent complications by watching for fever or malaise, which may signal the onset of infection; also check for signs of other problems, such as severe anemia and fractures. If the patient's bedridden, change his position every 2 hours. Perform passive range-of-motion exercises and instruct him to do deep-breathing exercises; when he can tolerate them, promote active range-of-motion exercises.
- Assess the patient daily for signs of increasing tumor mass, particularly in the spinal area.
- If the patient's receiving melphalan, make sure his blood count (platelet and WBC) is taken before each treatment. If he's taking prednisone, watch closely for infection, since this drug may mask it.
- Whenever possible, get the patient out of bed within 24 hours after laminectomy. Check for hemorrhage, motor or sensory deficits, and loss of bowel or bladder function. Position the patient as ordered, maintain alignment, and logroll when turning.
- Teach the patient how to recognize signs and symptoms of infection, spontaneous bone fractures, renal failure, and increasing tumor mass.
- Provide emotional support for the patient and his family. To alleviate their anxiety, truthfully inform them about diagnostic tests (including painful procedures, such as bone marrow aspiration and biopsy), treatment, and prognosis. If needed, refer them to an appropriate community resource for additional support.

Continued on page 150

Plasma Cell and Other Disorders

Plasma cell myeloma—*continued*

Evaluation

Base your evaluation on the expected outcomes listed on the nursing care plan. To determine whether your patient has improved, ask yourself the following questions:

- Does the patient state that he has pain?
- Can he tell you what intensifies or relieves his pain?
- Does he express pain relief?

The answers to these questions will help you evaluate your patient's status and the effectiveness of his care. Keep in mind that these questions stem from the sample care plan on page 147. Your questions may differ.

Other plasma cell disorders

Waldenström's macroglobulinemia

In Waldenström's macroglobulinemia (WM), also called primary macroglobulinemia, plasma B cell clones overproduce high-molecular-weight immunoglobulins in response to an antigenic signal. The abnormal immunoglobulins proliferate uncontrollably while normal immunoglobulin synthesis decreases. Most patients with WM have chromosomal abnormalities, such as a large median or submedian marker chromosome in peripheral blood lymphocytes, cell structure abnormalities, and abnormal chromosome levels.

WM sometimes occurs with amyloidosis, nonlymphoid cancers, rheumatoid arthritis, ankylosing spondylitis, Sjögren's syndrome, and acute leukemia. Although the disease's cause remains unknown, it frequently clusters in families. It most commonly affects older men.

WM may be accompanied by hyperviscosity syndrome, which can precipitate or exacerbate CHF. Visual disturbances—including hemorrhages, exudates, and venous congestion with vascular segmentation (sausage formation)—may be the most obvious signs.

WM can cause an increased infection rate and recurrent infections, typically with *Pneumocystis carinii* pneumonia and cytomegalic inclusion disease. Bleeding disorders, possibly related to hyperviscosity, may cause abnormal platelet adhesion, prothrombin time, and thromboplastin generation and a subnormal Factor VIII value.

About one third of WM patients experience renal failure. IgM deposits on the basement membrane's endothelium may block the capillary lumen and mimic thrombi. Most of these patients have lymphocytic or plasma cell infiltration. Amyloid deposits sometimes develop in the glomerulus. Dehydration may precipitate acute renal failure. Occasionally, patients have nephrotic syndrome (from deposition of monoclonal IgM with high-titer glomerular autoantibodies on the basement membrane).

Pulmonary involvement can occur in the form of diffuse infiltrates, isolated masses (consisting of plasmacytoid lymphocytes), or pleural effusion.

Although uncommon, diarrhea or steatorrhea may complicate WM. These problems may stem from monoclonal IgM deposition or lym-

Plasma Cell and Other Disorders

Waldenström's macroglobulinemia: Assessment findings

- Abnormal bleeding and purpura
- Congestive heart failure
- Fatigue and weakness
- Hepatomegaly
- Lymphadenopathy
- Neurologic abnormalities
- Raynaud's phenomenon (intermittent ischemic attacks of the fingers or toes, marked by pallor and sometimes paresthesia and pain)
- Splenomegaly
- Visual disturbances and ocular changes
- Weight loss

phocyte and plasma cell infiltration of the GI tract. IgM deposits also may affect the orbital and lacrimal glands.

Assessment. Because WM commonly causes bleeding, your patient may have a recent history of epistaxis, GI bleeding, dependent purpura, or other obvious or occult bleeding. With neurologic involvement, blurred vision, severely reduced visual acuity, or other neurologic symptoms can occur.

Your patient may also report hypersensitivity to cold, symptoms of Raynaud's phenomenon, urticaria, or purpura—possibly associated with cryoglobulinemia.

When performing the physical examination, you may detect liver and spleen enlargement, superficial lymph node enlargement, and retinal abnormalities. Dilated, tortuous retinal veins are the earliest retinal changes detectable by funduscopy. Sausagelike segmentation of distended retinal veins and retinal hemorrhages appear as hyperviscosity worsens. Erythrocyte clumping and venocapillary segmentation may occur in conjunctival vessels. A patient with marked hyperviscosity may suffer confusion, level of consciousness changes progressing to coma, and a diffuse brain syndrome known as *coma paraproteinaemicum.*

Also assess the patient for signs of neurologic abnormalities, including peripheral neuropathy, encephalopathy, a Guillain-Barré–like syndrome, and intracerebral or subarachnoid hemorrhage. Occasionally the initial sign of WM, peripheral neuropathy typically involves both sensory and motor function. Other neurologic problems may include auditory and vestibular dysfunction and progressive spinal muscular atrophy. Bing-Neel syndrome—WM accompanied by encephalopathy—may also occur.

Be sure to assess your patient's fluid balance. Markedly increased plasma volume, hyperviscosity, and anemia may cause CHF—an important complication with uncontrolled disease. Also check for respiratory abnormalities.

Diagnostic tests. These findings suggest WM:
- hemoglobin level of less than 12 g/dl
- relative serum viscosity of more than 4
- Bence Jones proteinemia
- decreased platelet adhesion, prothrombin time, and thromboplastin generation
- below-normal Factor VIII level
- increased plasma and mast cell levels in bone marrow
- cryoglobulin level of more than 3 g/dl and precipitate formation at room temperature, resulting in cold hypersensitivity
- positive Sia test (a drop of serum added to distilled water causes a precipitate cloud to form at the bottom of the container).

Intervention. Some patients with WM respond to treatment with chlorambucil, cyclophosphamide, prednisone, or melphalan. For a patient who has become refractory to alkylating agents, the doctor may order doxorubicin (Adriamycin).

A patient *without* the following signs may require only close observation: enlarged superficial lymph nodes, hepatosplenomegaly,

Continued on page 152

Plasma Cell and Other Disorders

Other plasma cell disorders—*continued*

bone lesions, anemia, bleeding tendencies, renal insufficiency, hyperviscosity, or neurologic changes. Such a patient may remain stable for years, never needing treatment. However, he should have regular checkups; if he shows a progressively increasing IgM concentration or becomes symptomatic, expect the doctor to order therapy.

A patient with hyperviscosity syndrome may require special treatment. For a patient with severe symptoms, the doctor will order plasmapheresis to remove 4 to 6 units of plasma daily until the relative serum viscosity drops below 4. Chemotherapy (chlorambucil or cyclophosphamide with prednisone), which controls the underlying disease, helps prevent recurrent hyperviscosity.

Heavy-chain diseases

These rare disorders are characterized by plasma cell tumors that produce immunoglobulin variants, usually consisting of separate defective heavy chains (incomplete molecules) with internal deletions. They're typically accompanied by ineffective light-chain synthesis. Two major types of heavy-chain diseases exist—gamma and alpha. (For information on less common heavy-chain diseases, see *Other heavy-chain diseases.*)

Gamma heavy-chain disease affects mostly persons over age 40 but can occur in those as young as age 12. Disease progression varies, with survival ranging from several months to 5 years or more; a few patients have complete remissions. Death usually results from infection or disease progression. Occasionally, patients develop terminal plasma cell leukemia.

Alpha heavy-chain disease is the most common form. Its incidence peaks in persons between ages 10 and 30. Two clinical disease forms exist:

- the enteric form (also known as Mediterranean lymphoma), concentrated in Mediterranean, Asian, and South American countries—areas with a high incidence of intestinal infection with parasites, bacteria, and viruses
- the respiratory form, seen mostly in Americans and Europeans, characterized by a lymphoplasmacytic infiltrate confined to the respiratory tract.

In most cases, alpha heavy-chain disease takes a progressive and fatal course, but complete remission can occur, as indicated by the disappearance of proteins from the serum and jejunal fluid and of lymphoplasmacytic infiltrate from the intestinal mucosa.

Assessment. Suspect gamma heavy-chain disease if your patient complains of fever, malaise, and weakness, possibly indicating anemia. The physical examination may reveal mild lymphadenopathy, especially in Waldeyer's ring (lymphoid tissue encircling the lingual, pharyngeal, and palatine tonsils). Palpable lymph nodes frequently wax and wane. You may also detect liver and spleen enlargement.

With enteric alpha heavy-chain disease, the patient may have a history of abdominal pain, chronic diarrhea, severe malabsorption with marked weight loss, steatorrhea, hypocalcemia, and excessive

Plasma Cell and Other Disorders

Other heavy-chain diseases

Mu heavy-chain disease. The few known patients with this disease, ranging from age 39 to 79, have had chronic lymphocytic leukemia (CLL) or another lymphoid neoplasm. Assessment findings include liver and spleen enlargement and, in a few cases, enlarged peripheral lymph nodes. Bone marrow commonly contains unusual vacuolated plasma cells (similar cells rarely appear in other plasma cell dyscrasias). Most patients have high urine levels of kappa light chains.

Immunoelectrophoresis usually shows a rapidly migrating component that precipitates with antisera to mu chains but not with antisera to light chains; free kappa chains of different mobility commonly appear. Ultracentrifugation or gel filtration is usually needed to further document the diagnosis. Bence Jones proteinemia occurs in most cases; however, mu chains rarely appear in the urine.

Expect the doctor to treat mu heavy-chain disease by treating the underlying problem (usually CLL). Patients typically have a prolonged survival.

Delta heavy-chain disease. Doctors have reported only one case of this disease. The patient had renal insufficiency, osteolytic lesions, and marrow plasmacytosis typical of myeloma. Electrophoresis revealed a peak of 700 mg/dl between the gamma and beta regions; a monoclonal delta tetramer appeared in the serum. The patient, who died of renal failure, had a glomerular accumulation of delta heavy-chain complexes.

electrolyte loss. You may detect palpable abdominal masses and finger clubbing.

Diagnostic tests. Diagnosis of gamma heavy-chain disease rests on serum and urine analysis supported by bone marrow, lymph node, and spleen biopsy findings. The serum, urine, or both contain a protein component that reacts with antisera to the gamma heavy chain but not with antisera to kappa or lambda light chains or Fab fragments.

Electrophoresis usually shows the abnormal protein as a heterogeneous band; serum and urine proteins have identical mobility. The abnormal protein may be nearly undetectable, or its concentration may reach 3 g/dl, with urinary excretion as high as 15 g/day.

Bone marrow biopsy typically shows increased plasma cell, lymphocyte, lymphocytoid plasma cell, and eosinophil levels. However, marrow findings rarely aid diagnosis. Spleen and lymph node biopsies usually show plasma cell or lymphocyte infiltration, sometimes accompanied by eosinophil and macrophage infiltration. Although pathology findings may resemble those of chronic lymphocytic leukemia or multiple myeloma, signs of lymphoid malignancy are rare.

With alpha heavy-chain disease, intestinal mucosal biopsy shows diffuse, massive lymphoplasmacytic infiltration of the lamina propria. Cell appearance ranges from normal plasma cells to immunoblastic sarcoma cells; atrophied villi and sparse crypts are also common. Mesenteric lymph node and rectal biopsies reveal comparable lymphoplasmacytic infiltration. In late disease, a tumor may obstruct the intestine. Bowel wall thickening, villous atrophy, and lymph node enlargement may appear on radiologic examination.

Lymphangiography sometimes shows enlarged retroperitoneal nodes but rarely reveals peripheral lymph node, liver, spleen, or skeletal involvement. The serum of a terminally ill patient may contain abnormal plasma or lymphoid cells; marrow may contain abnormal plasma cells.

Immunochemical serum studies confirm alpha heavy-chain disease. For instance, serum electrophoresis usually demonstrates a reduced albumin level; moderate to marked hypogammaglobulinemia; and a wide nonhomogeneous band in the beta$_2$- to alpha$_2$-globulin region, with a concentration from several hundred mg/dl to 3 g/dl.

Intervention. Treatment for gamma heavy-chain disease resembles treatment for PCM—drug therapy (such as with melphalan and cyclophosphamide) and local radiation therapy. For a patient with alpha heavy-chain disease, the doctor may order a chemotherapy regimen similar to those used to treat lymphoma, or he may order antibiotics alone. Such treatment has achieved remission in some patients.

Monocyte and macrophage disorders

Histiocytosis

In this disorder, histiocytes proliferate abnormally. Lesions typically contain sheetlike masses of proliferated histiocytes with many

Continued on page 154

Plasma Cell and Other Disorders

Monocyte and macrophage disorders—*continued*

eosinophils interspersed singly or in clusters. Histiocytes merge to form multinucleated giant cells; in some cases, vacuolated histiocyte aggregates exist. Histiocytosis takes one of two forms:

- localized, involving one organ (such as solitary eosinophilic granuloma of bone and pulmonary eosinophilic granuloma)
- systemic, involving several organ systems.

Eosinophilic granuloma of bone, a benign disease, remains confined to skeletal bone. Usually one circumscribed osteolytic lesion develops, although some patients have two or more. The disease affects men and women equally and has the highest incidence in older children and adults of any age.

Systemic histiocytosis can range from a fulminating disease to a relatively benign one. Occurring at any age, it most commonly affects children around age 3. The disease may involve all organ systems.

Assessment. With eosinophilic granuloma of bone, expect the patient to complain of pain and swelling over the affected sites. A lesion causing spinal cord compression can result in neurologic problems, including weakness and paralysis. Bone fractures may also occur.

With systemic histiocytosis, findings include the following:

- skeletal bone lesions. Lytic lesions, the most common type, have a somewhat different distribution than in disease localized to bone, occurring in the sella turcica and sphenoid bone. The maxilla, the mandible, and upper extremity bones are more likely to be involved than in localized disease. Although bone lesions may cause fractures, they rarely cause other symptoms. However, if adjacent soft tissues become involved, complications may arise. For instance, maxillary and mandibular disease may cause dental problems (loose teeth; mouth ulcers; hypertrophied, friable gums). Sella turcica lesions can cause diabetes insipidus; mastoid and temporal bone involvement can cause chronic ear drainage.
- skin lesions. Usually papular, scaly, and erythematous, these lesions are occasionally eczematous or seborrheic. Ecchymoses or petechiae also can occur. Rarely, nodular infiltrates and xanthomatous-appearing lesions develop.
- pituitary abnormalities. Growth hormone deficiency—characterized by shortened stature, hyperprolactinemia, and hypogonadism—and diabetes insipidus can result from pituitary involvement.
- eye and ear abnormalities. Bulging eyes (proptosis) may be bilateral or unilateral. Temporal bone involvement causes chronic, nonpurulent drainage from the ears and granulomatous tissue in the external auditory canals.
- lung lesions. Extensive lesions may cause cor pulmonale. Spontaneous pneumothorax may also occur, sometimes providing the first clue to the disease.
- enlarged lymph nodes. Local lymphadenopathy, possibly the first sign of the disease, may become prominent as the disease spreads extensively.
- liver, spleen, and bone marrow lesions. Usually occurring simultaneously, these lesions signal a grave prognosis.

Plasma Cell and Other Disorders

Diagnostic tests. Laboratory studies usually aren't sufficient to diagnose localized histiocytosis. However, localized pulmonary eosinophilic granuloma appears on a chest X-ray as a diffuse, interstitial, nodular infiltrate with small cystic areas arranged in a honeycomb pattern. Pulmonary function studies may reveal an alveolocapillary blockage. Lung biopsy confirms pulmonary eosinophilic granuloma. With systemic histiocytosis, leukocytosis may appear, but bone marrow biopsy and other studies appear normal.

Intervention. For eosinophilic granuloma of bone, the doctor may order a biopsy followed by curettage and radiation therapy. Most patients respond well and have an excellent prognosis. (However, in some cases, bone lesions are the first sign of systemic histiocytosis or precede other lesions—especially in children.) Pulmonary eosinophilic granuloma usually responds well to glucocorticoid and radiation therapy.

Systemic histiocytosis may respond to glucocorticoids, antibiotics, radiation therapy, and various cytotoxic and antimetabolite agents. Radiation's typically used to treat specific local problems, such as bone lesions predisposing to fracture or chronically draining ears. Vasopressin (Pitressin), given parenterally or by inhalation, controls diabetes insipidus.

Gaucher's disease

An autosomal recessive disorder, Gaucher's disease is characterized by an abnormal accumulation of glucocerebrosides (lipid substances containing a glucose sugar) in monocytes and macrocytes. It occurs in three forms:

- Type I (adult), the most common form; most prevalent among Jews of European origin. (*Note:* Type I disease is usually diagnosed while the patient's in his teens; the word adult is used loosely here.)
- Type II (infantile)
- Type III (juvenile).

The spleen may become extremely enlarged, and splenic sequestration may cause hemolysis, leukopenia, and severe thrombocytopenia. The liver may also become enlarged; hepatic fibrosis and esophageal varices may develop. Severe pulmonary disease, characterized by cyanosis and clubbed fingers, occurs in some patients with liver involvement. Glucocerebroside accumulation in bone can cause localized bone destruction. The femur—the most commonly involved bone—may become swollen, especially around the head and neck of the bone.

Assessment. With Type I disease, the patient may complain of severe episodic pain in the legs, arms, and back; fever; and easy bruising. When performing the physical examination, check for liver and spleen enlargement, bone lesions (possibly causing pathologic fractures, collapsed hip joints, and vertebral compression), abdominal distention, respiratory problems (pneumonia or, rarely, cor pulmonale), yellow pallor, and brown-yellow pigmentation on the face and legs.

With Type II disease, motor dysfunction and spasticity occur at age 6 to 7 months. Other signs include abdominal distention, strabismus, muscular hypertonicity, retroflexion of the head, neck ri-

Continued on page 156

Plasma Cell and Other Disorders

Monocyte and macrophage disorders—*continued*

gidity, dysphagia, laryngeal stridor, hyperreflexia, seizures, respiratory distress, and easy bruising and bleeding. Clinical effects of Type III disease include seizures, hypertonicity, strabismus, poor coordination and mental ability, and, possibly, easy bruising and bleeding.

Diagnostic tests. Expect the doctor to order a bone marrow biopsy (which shows Gaucher cells) and direct assay of glucocerebrosidase activity. Supportive laboratory test results include an increased serum acid phosphatase level and decreased platelet, leukocyte, and serum iron levels. Type I disease commonly includes anemia and, rarely, pancytopenia. In Type III disease, an EEG done after infancy is abnormal.

Intervention. Treatment's mainly supportive and consists of vitamins, supplemental iron or liver extract to prevent anemia caused by iron deficiency and to alleviate other hematologic problems, blood transfusions for anemia, splenectomy for thrombocytopenia, and strong analgesics for bone pain.

Nursing intervention.
- If the patient's confined to bed, prevent pathologic fractures by turning him carefully. If he's ambulatory, see that he's assisted when getting out of bed or walking.
- Observe the patient closely for changes in pulmonary status.
- Help the patient and/or his family accept the limitations imposed by this disorder.
- Recommend genetic counseling for parents who want to have another child.

Self-Test

1. Which of the following is the most common sign of Hodgkin's disease?
a. Pel-Ebstein fever **b.** persistent cough **c.** pruritus
d. painless cervical lymphadenopathy

2. If your patient tests positive for AIDS with the ELISA test, it means he definitely has the disease. True or False?
a. True **b.** False

3. What is the hallmark of plasma cell myloma?
a. hypercalciuria **b.** Bing-Neel syndrome **c.** Bence Jones protein
d. hypercalcemia

4. Baby Smith has been diagnosed as having Gaucher's disease. Which type does he have?
a. Type I **b.** Type II **c.** Type III **d.** Type IV

Answers (page number shows where answer appears in text)
1. **d** (page 120) 2. **b** (pages 136 and 137) 3. **c** (pages 144 and 146) 4. **b** (page 155)

Selected References

Books

Alspach, JoAnn G., and Williams, Susan M., eds. *Core Curriculum for Critical Care Nursing,* 3rd ed. Philadelphia: W.B. Saunders Co., 1985.

Beck, William S., ed. *Hematology,* 3rd ed. Cambridge, Mass.: The MIT Press, 1983.

Brown, Barbara A. *Hematology: Principles and Procedures,* 4th ed. Philadelphia: Lea & Febiger, 1984.

Brown, Mary H., et al. *Standards of Oncology Nursing Practice.* New York: John Wiley and Sons, 1986.

Brunner, Lillian, and Suddarth, Doris. *The Lippincott Manual of Nursing Practice,* 4th ed. Philadelphia: J.B. Lippincott Co., 1986.

DeVita, Vincent, et al. *Cancer: Principles and Practice of Oncology,* 2nd ed. Philadelphia: J.B. Lippincott Co., 1985.

Fishbach, Frances T. *A Manual of Laboratory Diagnostic Tests,* 2nd ed. Philadelphia: J.B. Lippincott Co., 1984.

Griffin, Joyce P. *Hematology and Immunology: Concepts for Nursing.* East Norwalk, Conn.: Appleton and Lange, 1986.

Hamilton, Helen K., and McVan, Barbara F., eds. *Diseases* (Nurse's Reference Library), 2nd ed. Springhouse, Pa.: Springhouse Corporation, 1987.

Kirkpatrick, Constance S. *Nurse's Guide to Cancer Care.* Totowa, N.J.: Rowman and Littlefield, 1986.

Luckmann, Joan, and Sorensen, Karen C. *Medical-Surgical Nursing: A Psychophysiologic Approach,* 3rd ed. Philadelphia: W.B. Saunders Co., 1987.

McNally, Joan, et al., eds. *Guidelines for Cancer Nursing Practice.* Orlando, Fla.: Grune and Stratton, Inc., 1985.

O'Connor, Barbara H. *A Color Atlas and Instruction Manual of Peripheral Blood Morphology.* Baltimore, Md.: Williams and Wilkins, 1984.

Patrick, Maxine, et al. *Medical-Surgical Nursing: Pathophysiological Concepts.* Philadelphia: J.B. Lippincott Co., 1986.

Pittiglio, D. Harmening, ed. *Clinical Hematology and Fundamentals of Hemostasis.* Philadelphia: F.A. Davis & Co., 1987.

Rifkind, Richard A., et al. *Fundamentals of Hematology,* 3rd ed. Chicago: Yearbook Medical Publishers, 1986.

Serjeant, Graham R. *Sickle Cell Disease.* New York: Oxford University Press, Inc., 1985.

Spivak, Jerry L., ed. *Fundamentals of Clinical Hematology,* 2nd ed. Philadelphia: J.B. Lippincott Co., 1983.

Thompson, June M., et al. *Clinical Nursing.* St. Louis: C.V. Mosby Co., 1986.

Weiss, Harvey J., ed. *Platelets: Pathophysiology and Antiplatelet Drug Therapy.* New York: Alan R. Liss, Inc., 1984.

Williams, William J., et al. *Hematology,* 3rd ed. New York: McGraw-Hill Book Co., 1983.

Young, N., and Speck, B. *Aplastic Anemia: Stem Cell Biology and Advances in Treatment.* (Progress in Clinical and Biological Research Series, vol. 148). New York: Alan R. Liss, Inc., 1984.

Periodicals

Conant, M.A., et al. "Confronting AIDS in Primary Care," *Patient Care* 21(11):18-38, June 1987.

Foote, Michelle. "Nursing Care of the Patient with Non-Hodgkin's Lymphoma: Prevention of Pneumonia Associated with Combination Chemotherapy," *Cancer Nursing* 8(5):263-271, October 1985.

Gale, R., and Champlin, R. "Bone Marrow Transplantation in Acute Leukemia," *Clinics in Haematology* 15(3):851-868, 1986.

Griffin, Joyce P. "Nursing Care of the Critically Ill Cancer Patient with Cardiopulmonary Failure," *Critical Care Quarterly* 9(1):35-39, 1986.

Siegrist, Carl W., and Jones, Joyce A. "Disseminated Intravascular Coagulopathy and Nursing Implications," *Seminars in Oncology Nursing* 1(4):237-243, November 1985.

Terry, B.A. "Hodgkin's Disease and Non-Hodgkin's Lymphomas," *Nursing Clinics of North America* 20(1):207-217, March 1985.

Index

i refers to an illustration; t to a table; c to a chart.

Index

i refers to an illustration; t to a table; c to a chart.

Index

i refers to an illustration; t to a table; c to a chart.